COMMUNITY SYSTEMS AND HUMAN SERVICES

An Ecological Approach to Policy, Planning, and Management

Drew Hyman
Joe A. Miller

Department of Community Studies
College of Human Development
The Pennsylvania State University

Kendall/Hunt
Publishing Company
Dubuque, Iowa

This edition has been printed directly from camera-ready copy.

Copyright © 1985 by Kendall/Hunt Publishing Company

Library of Congress Catalog Card Number: 84–52586

ISBN 0–8403–4001–X

Second Printing, 1986

Printed in the United States of America

B   404001   02

"NEW ANSWERS MUST BE FOUND BY US.
THEY MUST BE WORKED OUT NOT ONLY
IN THE QUIET CONTEMPLATION OF THE STUDY,
BUT IN THE DUST AND SWEAT,
THE SWIRL AND THUNDER
OF THE ARENA.
AND THEY MUST BE, ABOVE ALL,
DISPASSIONATE--DETERMINED NOT
BY THE PREJUDICES WE BRING
TO A PROBLEM,
BUT BY THE FACTS
WE FIND IN IT."

-Robert Kennedy

CONTENTS

PREFACE

"This notion of community is one of the most characteristic, one of the most important, yet one of the least noticed American contributions to modern life. . . . In America, even in modern times, communities existed before governments were here to care for public needs. There were many groups of people with a common sense of purpose and a feeling of duty to one another before there were political institutions forcing them to perform their duties."

—Daniel Boorstin*

This book is about systems, policy and community services. It also addresses issues of planning, organizing, implementation and management. It is most specifically about the highly complex structures and interactions in American communities which we call "human service systems." The social and institutional networks in which these systems exist encompass the public and private sectors of our society. They are influenced, and often organized by government policies at state and local, federal and regional levels. They address issues of health, justice, social and economic well-being, child welfare, mental health, housing, transportation, aging, urban planning and community development.

Human service systems exist in all of our communities. They surround us. They extend into our lives daily. We, our neighbors, and thousands of others contribute to their problems, operation and performance. The interactions of these social institutions with communities, and the effects they have on our lives, well-being and quality of life are frequent and pervasive.

----

* Daniel J. Boorstin, "From Charity to Philanthropy," in America's Voluntary Spirit, Brian O'Connel, ed. N.Y.: The Foundation Center, 1983, p. 131.

Throughout the book you will be asked to consider the policies and processes through which communities plan, organize, and manage human services, and how human services improve and complicate our lives.

Six key concepts which permeate our discussion--"systems," "community," "policy," "planning," "management," and "human services"--are among the most elusive in our contemporary vocabulary. They mean many things to many people. They are often used indiscriminately to describe a wide variety of phenomena The first objective of the book is to "tune-in" to these terms. The concepts are explicated in a design to enable you to synthesize material from this book with knowledge and experience you gain from other sources. You are asked to read, to observe, to contemplate, and to integrate material from your personal experiences and knowledge of community to make this book meaningful and useful to you.

Our second, and equally important objective is to provide beginning professionals in human development fields with a basic understanding of the organization and dynamics of human services systems and programs. More specifically, our focus is on the deliberative processes of planning, organizing, implementing, and managing through which social policies originate and are subsequently translated into programs and delivery systems that make services available to individuals and groups at the local community level. Thus, we emphasize the ends (policies) and the means (programs) of purposive efforts to help citizens, individually and collectively, deal with problems of daily living. At the same time, we stress the local community because this is the setting in which such problems experienced by individuals and groups intersect with policies and programs designed to serve their needs--or, as is true in many instances, where the primary impact of a disjuncture between problems and sources of help is experienced.

With these brief introductory comments in mind, we can state that our plan for this book is to help you, the reader, to attain three important learning objectives:

o   To develop a working knowledge of social policies and programs as planned interventions to assist individuals, families, neighborhoods, and entire local communities in dealing with problems affecting the quality of life and daily patterns of living.

o   To develop a working knowledge of "systems" as an essential organizing concept for analyzing and assessing community policies and programs--i.e.. why some work very well and others do not, and what might be done to improve their effectiveness, whether at the policy, administrative or service delivery levels.

o   To develop a working knowledge of how social policies and programs are planned, organized, and managed at national, state, and local levels--whether in the public (governmental) or private (non-governmental) sectors.

Although the book is intended to be a practical guide to understanding policies and programs in the general field of community and human services, it does not ignore important theoretical and conceptual issues underlying these key concerns. As we move along from chapter to chapter, you will be introduced to many conceptual and theoretical terms that we regard as essential in learning to analyze policies and programs as planned interventions for individual and community development. Some of these, such as "policy," "program," "human services," "community" and "systems" are absolutely necessary to a systematic understanding of how policies come into being and are implemented in the United States. Moreover, to understand current policies and programs, it is important to see how societal values and orientations to human development issues have emerged over time. Furthermore, for the practising human development professional, whatever the specific field of employment, a basis for interpreting current trends that appear to be influencing patterns of social policy into the future is an important concern.

In setting our objectives for the book, we have made very few assumptions about the background any reader might have in the area of social policies and programs. Although the terms "system," "policy," "community," and "human services" are very common parts of our everyday vocabularies, we have assumed that, for most readers, the concepts will have rather hazy or unclear meanings when it comes to specific applications. For example, most people will have some vague understanding, at least, that federal, state and local governments have "welfare policies" that define types and levels of public assistance to low-income individuals and families who are unable to take care of their own needs--whether these needs arise from old age, unemployment of a family's main wage earner, or physical disability. Fewer people will associate what they have heard about "price supports" for farmers selling their crops in the marketplace with federal social (and economic) policy to maintain adequate individual and family incomes for a particular occupational group. Additionally, most of us will be aware that governments today are attempting to mprove the quality of air we breathe through legislation requiring unleaded gasoline and pollution control devices in all new automobiles, imposing regulations concerned with the release of impurities into the air from fuel-burning factories, or preventing chemical manufacturers from dumping waste materials into public waterways. All of these, and many thousands of other examples that could be presented, are examples of social policies. Together, they begin to illustrate the extent to which our daily lives are affected by social policies and programs at all levels of the American community.

As the succeeding chapters will show, our primary emphasis is on social policies and programs that are planned and delivered to individuals, families, social groups and entire communities in local settings. This, however, does not mean that our discussion will ignore extralocal policy and planning systems for human development. Such systems at state and national levels, both governmental and non-governmental in form, are often the sources of policy guidelines and financial support for services ultimately delivered at the local community level. An understanding of how these different system levels interrelate--as an intergovernmental system in the public sector or as a hierarchically based corporate system in the non-governmental (private) sector--is essential for interpreting which services are made available to citizens in their local communities.

In moving on to the main chapters of this book we wish to emphasize that our discussion will not encompass the entire field of social policies and programs. That would be an impossible task, given the thousands of policies and programs to be found in the governmental and non-governmental sectors. Rather, we shall be pursuing the more general goal of providng the reader with a **general** framework that can be used in analyzing particular social policies, community systems, and human services.

We wish to thank our former students in Community Development (now Community Studies) in the College of Human Development at Penn State for teaching us about which concepts, theories and perspectives are most important to the entering professional. Both those who have entered the field as workers in community systems and those who have gone on to professional graduate programs stressed the importance of a fundamental understanding of systems and their application in community and human service policies and programs. We hope we have been true to their "feedback" in presenting this text as an orientation to these issues. We also learned from them about the importance of applying theories and concepts to "real-world" situations. We hope that the many examples, case situations, and illustrations facilitate not only the understanding of concepts, but also their application in the field.

We also wish to thank our families, in particular Donna Hyman and Nancy Miller, for their patience and advice, and above all their critical reading of portions of the text as they were prepared. Donna's background in human services, and Nancy's experience in editing provided for reality-testing of both form and content as the book developed. We also wish to thank Kelly Hyman for her diligence in word processing of the many drafts, and for patience in the correction and revision process, and Stacy Hyman for preparation of the index. Finally, the support of our colleagues in the College of Human Development facilitated the development and production of the book. Ray Studer, Chairman of the Department of Community Studies, and J. Gregory Carroll, Associate Dean for Instruction, in particular, provided encouragement and support at key phases. Now let us move to consideration of the many facets of the kaleidoscopic system of which we are a part.

University Park, Pa.

x

Chapter I

WHAT IT'S ALL ABOUT: PERSPECTIVES ON COMMUNITY SYSTEMS AND HUMAN SERVICES

"Nothing endures but change."
–Heraclitus

"Our little systems have their day."
–Alfred, Lord Tennyson

Opening Comments

This book is about policies and planning for programs and services in human development. More pointedly, we are principally concerned with community environments and the many different human service systems that are found in these local settings.

We envision our typical reader as someone who is currently engaged in basic professional education for eventual employment in a human services agency or organization. This may involve specialized training to become a counselor or probation officer in the youth services field, a nurse practitioner or nutritionist in an institutional setting or a community agency, a planning analyst in a local economic or social development organization, or an administrative trainee in a voluntary or proprietary health services organization--a few examples of the myriad jobs encompassed by the general label of "human services." This book deals with only a few facets of this professional preparation but important ones, nonetheless.

Regardless of the particular human services setting in which our typical reader-student may subsequently be employed--most likely, starting out in an entry-level, "front-line" position--the effects of policies and programmatic guidelines will permeate daily professional activities. This will be equally true for those working in positions of direct client contact and for others in jobs involving work with planning data and information, rather than directly meeting with individual clients or client groups. Such constraints are simply a fact of professional life.

As we continue to move through the decade of the 1980s, staying alert to changes in social policies and programs is a vital concern for all human service professionals. For example, recent cutbacks in support by the federal government for domestic social programs has resulted in a shrinkage of resources for human services at all levels of society--national, state, and local. For those who work in local environments, it is a time for ingenuity in the planning, management, and delivery of community human services.

An important ingredient of such ingenuity is the ability to apply critical thinking to the concepts and principles that underlie the essence of social policies and programs in human services and human development. Macarov, in commenting on essential skills for social workers in the future, has noted that professional effectiveness will require a **combination** of conceptual and technical skills: "The use of concepts is an indication of critical thinking, and it is critical thinking, not mere technical ability, that will mark the competent social worker of the future." (1978, page 8) Macarov's trenchant comments about the "competent social worker" of the future can, **de facto,** be applied to the entire range of human service professions.

A systematic understanding of the essential characteristics of social policies and programs, their planning and management, and their delivery in local community settings is a fundamental ingredient of basic professional education for the human services. This book is dedicated to helping each reader develop a working knowledge of these vital concerns.

Objectives of This Chapter

This chapter has three major objectives. Each is concerned with helping our readers begin to understand the nature and functions of social policies and programs in relation to human development needs and human services delivery.

o   Our **first** objective is to help each reader establish a personal perspective on the varied types of needs and helping services subsumed by the general label of "human services." We do this through the presentation of a series of brief case descriptions of different types of human development problems and various human services that may be brought to bear on each situation.

o   Our **second** objective is to introduce a basic vocabulary of concepts and terminology that will be discussed in greater detail in later chapters of the book. Our purpose here is to help each reader to begin to get a "feel" for the concepts and themes that are essential to the development of a working knowledge of social policies and programs, especially as these are manifest at a community systems level.

o   Our **third** objective is to present a case review of a social policy area which has become increasingly relevant to community human service concerns in recent decades. For this purpose, we have chosen the topic of employment and training programs. This, we feel, is a very practical choice at a time when increasing numbers of workers are experiencing the impact of permanent job loss through plant shutdowns and shifts in corporate preferences for industrial locations from the "Frostbelt" areas of the Northeast and Upper Midwest to the "Sunbelt" regions of the Southern, Southwestern, and Western United States.

>>As each objective is unfolded in this chapter, ask yourself the following questions. First, what is the scope of "human services" and "human development"? Second, what concepts and principles are essential to understand the impact of social policies on **community** human services? Third, how do different hierarchical levels of legislative and/or corporate authority influence the planning, management, and delivery of **local** human services?<<

Getting Down to Cases

Social policy and planning for community human services are, admittedly, pretty broad areas of subject matter. Where to begin one's understanding of what it is all about is an important question.

There are two quite different ways to start wrestling with the subject. One is to begin with concepts, definitions, and principles, and then move on to see how these might be applied to practical problems in human development. Another is to look first at some practical examples of human development problems and attempt to see how they might be connected to policy and program concerns.

We have chosen the latter method for this opening chapter. This is not because we are uninterested in abstract concepts or general principles--or, for that matter, definitions. Our interest in these and our concern that our readers learn about them and how to apply them will be evident throughout this book. We believe strongly that the ability to blend the general and the particular--that is, dealing with specific problems by applying general concepts and principles--is the hallmark of the well-trained human development professional.

Below, we present several brief case descriptions. Each represents a different type of practical problem experienced by an individual or group--two basic entities with which we are ultimately concerned when we refer to "human development." We've included a variety of problem situations in these vignettes to help you get a feel for the broad range of circumstances that are covered by social policies and programs for human development and human services.

o   John S. has been employed as an engineer in the XYZ Corporation for almost 12 years. Lately, he has been feeling strained by the pressures of his job--in fact, rather useless and "burnt out." To try to deal with his stress, he has begun to drink heavily, which has not only affected his productivity on the job but also his relations with co-workers. Recently, John's supervisor confronted him about his deteriorating productivity and the strained relationships he was creating throughout his work group. He noted that John was a valued employee of the corporation and that he would hate to see disciplinary action become necessary. He recommended that John get in touch with the XYZ Corporation's "Employee Assistance Program" (EAP) to get help with his problems. John followed up on his supervisor's suggestion and became a participant in his employer's EAP.

o   Mrs. Oliver is an 80-year old widow. Her husband died several years ago, leaving her alone in the family house which is well over 50 years old and badly in need of upkeep. Never having worked herself, she receives a modest monthly Social Security check as her husband's survivor. A neighbor notices that Mrs. Oliver apparently has no friends, eats very little and then not a balanced diet, and spends nearly all of her time alone watching television. The neighbor gets in touch with the County's local Area Agency on Aging, which contacts Mrs. Oliver, arranging for her to enroll in the local Meals-on-Wheels program, for the local Home Health Service to send a chore worker to help with minor repairs to the house and its upkeep, and for the local Voluntary Action Center to have a volunteer home visitor to call at Mrs. Oliver's house

5

on a regular basis to provide her with companionship and assist her in getting out of the house from time to time to shop and attend programs at the local Senior Citizens Center.

o   Mr. Jones was laid off from his job several months ago. There is little chance that he will ever be asked to return to his former job, even though he had worked for the same employer for over 16 years. During the first several months, he received unemployment compensation checks from the state, which helped him and his family meet their income needs. He also attended and participated in the self-help "Job Club" sponsored by his former employer--learning how to prepare a personal resume, how to search for a new job, and how to "stretch the dollar" with his reduced income. Now, though his unemployment compensation has expired, he hasn't been able to find a new job and no longer has the health insurance fringe benefits that had been part of his old job to cover his family's doctor and medical bills. Mr. Jones, in desperate financial circumstances, goes to the local county board of assistance to seek public welfare help with his and his family's income and medical needs.

o   Mrs. Smith separated from her husband nine months ago but has received no support from him for their three children or herself. She is receiving public assistance through the Aid to Families with Dependent Children program but desperately needs new housing, since the home she and her husband owned was recently repossessed for nonpayment of the mortgage. She gets in touch with the local housing authority, which is able to help her through the "Section 8" housing assistance program for low-income families administered at the federal level by the Department of Housing and Urban Development and locally by the county's Public Housing Authority.

o   Mr. and Mrs. Brown have been married for 13 years and have two children. Lately, the pressures of Mrs. Brown's part-time job and her domestic work of cooking, laundering, housecleaning, ironing, and getting the kids off to school every morning--since Mr. Brown gives her little or no help with any of these--have led to an increasing number of rancorous arguments between the couple about parenting and the sharing of responsibilities at home. In fact, they both wonder if their marriage will survive or even whether it's worth saving. They try, though, to talk things out, and decide to begin meeting with a private marriage counselor on a weekly basis to see if they can get their marital problems straightened out and find ways to relieve some of the pressures felt by Mrs. Brown.

o   Many residents of a local neighborhood in a large metropolitan community have become very upset about the inreasing rates of vandalism, burglaries, and personal assaults in their residential area. They call a meeting of local residents to see what they might do themselves to deal with these problems. It is decided to organize a "crime watch" awareness program, using volunteers from among the residents. They also approach the City Council for help in organizing the neighborhood program and getting it underway. The City Council authorizes the use of funds and the services of the local police department to assist the neighborhood group in setting up the crime watch program and beginning its operation.

o   A medium-size city of 80,000 has been losing industries and jobs steadily over the past few years. Recently, a manufacturer of small airplanes announced that it would be closing its local plant because of declining sales, after being one of the city's major employers for nearly 50 years. The city council, working with the local Industrial Development

7

Authority (a local nonprofit corporation) begins to analyze systematically the city's economic and employment problems, with a view to drawing up a long-range plan for local economic revitalization and the generation of jobs by attracting new employers to their city. The plan calls for using local government's zoning and taxing authority to lay the groundwork for incentives to new business to locate in the city, and drawing upon the state's industrial loan program for local economic development. It also relies on the local Private Industry Council to help by implementing job training programs for the unemployed to give them job skills that will meet the needs of new businesses and industries that might decide to locate in the city.

Now, look back over these several brief case illustrations. What do they have in common and how do they differ?

First, each reflects an instance of individual or collective distress that requires outside help for a solution. Dealing with the problem is beyond the reach of the individual's or group's own resources.

Second, each case illustrates a problem concerned with material, physical, mental or social well-being. Such concerns are the essence of human development, regardless of the particular circumstance or concrete problem facing an individual or group.

Third, each case also demonstrates that multiple needs frequently interrelate to create the overall problem confronting an individual or a group. Consequently, such problems often require bringing the resources of **several** helping systems to bear, in order to arrive at effective solutions.

There are, of course, several differences in how the various problems were handled and the types of external helping resources drawn upon in trying to resolve them. In some instances, public agencies were the primary service delivery systems; for example, the Area Agency on Aging, the local housing authority, the public welfare assistance agency, and the state unemployment compensation program. In others, voluntary nonprofit organizations were the providers of services; for example, the local voluntary action center, the local home health agency, and the local industrial development corporation. In yet other instances, help was obtained from private sources, such as an employer-sponsored EAP and a private practitioner in family counseling.

Another difference among these case illustrations pertains to the target, or intervention, level of the helping services. In some of the cases, the services were directed to the needs of individuals and in others to families or other groups. In the case of the planned program for local industrial and economic development, the entire community is the intended beneficiary.

In sum, we use the concepts of **human development** and **human services** in reference to concerns with both individual and collective well-being. In doing so, we are employing general labels that encompass a broad range of specific circumstances, problems, and forms of service delivery. As we shall see throughout this book, "getting down to cases" is a much more complex matter than one might believe it to be, at least initially. Furthermore, most problems seldom come in simple, one-issue form. Learning to see how problems often interrelate and how solutions to them frequently require linking together several helping systems is one of the most critical challenges facing the beginning human development professional.

Let's now move on to consider some of the essential concepts and general perspectives pertaining to human services and social welfare that will help us begin to deal effectively with this complexity.

Establishing Boundaries

In any intellectual undertaking, establishing the boundaries of concern is an important first step. That is our general goal in the next several sections of this chapter. Our specific aims are twofold.

First, we wish to introduce some key issues and general concepts related to the planning and delivery of community human services. Each of the topics dealt with here will be considered in greater detail in later chapters. At this point, we wish only to introduce the reader to the basic contours of the conceptual terrain over which we shall be traveling in the rest of the book.

Second, we want the reader to get an initial grasp of terms and labels that are essential to a **critical** understanding of social policies and planning for community human services. Simply to know **what** a concept or term of reference means is insufficient for thinking critically about human development and social welfare concerns. It is also important to know **why** it is essential and **how** it can be applied critically and analytically to an issue of planning, management, or delivery of human services in local community settings.

Now, let's look at some of the key ingredients of terminology that identify the boundaries of our concern in this book.

Human Services and Social Welfare

The concept of **human services** is not easily defined. Morris (1977) comments that a part of the definitional issue arises from the fact that it is still an evolving conception regarding the provision of services designed to secure or improve the well-being of individuals and groups in society. On the one hand, it continues to be a label that includes what heretofore went under the general heading of "social welfare." On the other, it attempts to go beyond what some perceive as limitations of the social welfare concept by encompassing additional areas of concern with problems in human development.

The question of what does--or, perhaps, should--enter into a definition of the human services concept is dealt with in subsequent chapters (especially Chapter IV). Here, we would only note that an overlap of the concepts of **human services** and **social welfare,** although not complete, is indisputable. For example, Romanyshyn's definition of social welfare could, in our opinion, serve equally well if the term of reference was human services:

> A set of institutions and services to promote the well-being of the populations and the better functioning of the social order. It includes those provisions and processes directly concerned with the treatment and prevention of social problems, development of human resources, and

improvement in the quality of life. It involves social services to individuals and groups as well as efforts to strengthen or modify social institutions. (Romanyshyn, 1981)

Romanyshyn suggests that social welfare services are intended to be both ameliorative and preventative with respect to individual and collective problems in human development and daily living. This, we feel, is the essence of the human services concept, regardless of the specific problem addressed, provider system, or target population for services delivery.

Societal Orientations to the Provision of Human Services

Human services are directed toward the physical, material, mental and social needs of individuals and groups. How services are made available to those in need of outside help with their problems depends, to a great extent, on societal values regarding ideas of self-reliance and family responsibility, and other values pertaining to communal responsibilities toward those in need of helping services.
Such orientations to philanthropic and social welfare assistance have been described in several different ways. Here, we briefly review two such orientations simply to give a sense of the different value systems that influence the ways in which human services are allocated to populations differing in economic and social statuses.

Compassion and Protection

Pumphrey has suggested that compassion and protection can be viewed as dual motivations for philanthropic efforts to assist others with their individual and social needs. "Compassion and protection represent two more or less consciously determined purposes that may be served by any given philanthropic enterprise." (Pumphrey, 1959, page 22)
The motive of **compassion** can be depicted as "the effort to alleviate present suffering, deprivation, or other undesirable

conditions to which a segment of the population, but not the benefactor, is exposed." (Pumphrey, 1959, page 21) Thus, helping services deriving from compassionate motives are directed toward meeting obvious present needs, not to ways of preventing the underlying problem that created the onset of the need.

The other philanthropic motive, **protection,** is more concerned with the prevention of problems and behaviors that are considered detrimental to communal interests. According to Pumphrey, services stemming from this motivation are those "in which the promoters, not only on their own behalf, but on behalf of their group or of the whole community, endeavor to prevent unwanted developments." (Pumphrey, 1959, page 22) For example, Charles Loring Brace, who founded the New York Children's Aid society in 1853, was concerned about the protection of society from the "dangerous classes." He felt that the slum conditions in New York City were not only unhealthy environments in which to raise children but also, if neglected and left unreformed, were distinct threats to the social order of the larger community. Thus, he noted:

> Society must act on the highest principles, or its
> punishment incessantly comes within itself. The neglect
> of the poor, and tempted, and criminal, is fearfully repaid.
> (Brace, 1880)

In sum, as Pumphrey notes, the "basic distinction is that in compassion the benefactor identifies with and seeks to alleviate the present pain which another feels; in protection he guards against painful consequences to himself, his group, or his community in the future." (1959, pages 23-24)

Residual and Institutional

Several years ago, Wilensky and Lebeaux suggested two labels, residual and institutional, to depict dominant societal orientations to social welfare in the United States. They described each of these conceptions in the following way.

> The first [i.e., the residual] holds that social welfare
> institutions should come into play only when the normal

structures of supply, the family and the market, break down. The second [i.e., the institutional] . . . sees the welfare services as normal, 'first line' functions of modern industrial society.

The residual formulation is based on the premise that there are two 'natural' channels through which an individual's needs are properly met: the family and the market economy. . . . [The social welfare structure] is conceived as a residual agency, attending primarily to emergency functions, and is expected to withdraw when the regular social structure--the family and the economic system--is again working properly. Because of its residual, temporary, substitute characteristic, social welfare thus conceived often carries the stigma of 'dole' or 'charity.'

[The] definition of the 'institutional' view implies no stigma, no emergency, no 'abnormalcy.' Social welfare becomes accepted as a proper, legitimate function of modern industrial society in helping individuals achieve self-fulfillment. The complexity of modern life is recognized. (Wilensky and Lebeaux, 1958, pages 138-140)

Wilensky and Lebeaux's work has had a pervasive influence on others who have written about the history and development of human services in the United States. For example, it is widely noted that it was not until the dire economic conditions of the Great Depression era of the 1930s that the federal government began moving towards the institutionalization of social welfare services for the needy--the first major embodiment being the Social Security Act of 1935.*

----

* It must be remembered that, in the depths of the Depression years, upwards of one-fourth to one-third of the labor force in the United States was unemployed. None of the subsequent economic recessions of the late 1950s and 1970s, or the high rates of unemployment in the early 1980s comes close to matching the extent of economic and unemployment problems in the depths of the Great Depression years.

In the pre-1930 years, there was little commitment or sensitivity by the federal government towards the need for financial or other kinds of assistance for the elderly, other low-income groups, and the unemployed. In fact, throughout all three levels of government--federal, state, and local--there was great reluctance to accept public responsibility for problems which were viewed, on the one hand, as stemming from individual laziness or inefficiency, and on the other, as being properly taken care of by private charitable and philanthropic organizations.

Such orientations toward poverty and human needs reflected a widespread acceptance in the United States of the English welfare traditions, most thoroughly expressed in the Elizabethan Poor Laws of 1601. This tradition distinguished between the "deserving poor"-- which included people with physical or mental disabilities not of their own making, orphans, widows and deserted mothers with small children--and the "undeserving poor"--which included those who were regarded as capable of working but did not, often referred to in the language of the day as "sturdy beggars."

This residual view of the social welfare function was buttressed in the United States by another viewpoint regarding the proper role of government in the affairs of citizens. The dominant orientation throughout the 19th century and well into the 20th was that large-scale federal intervention was contradictory to the United States Constitution, which, or so it was held, provided no basis for such an assumption of power and authority by the federal government.

This viewpoint on the limited role of the federal government was most clearly expressed in the case of a bill passed by Congress in 1854, which would have authorized a land grant to the states of 10 million acres to be used to build institutions for the housing and care of the mentally ill and the blind. This was a piece of legislation that an avid reformer of this period, Dorothea Dix, had advocated for many years, having documented the poor, unsanitary conditions under which most of the mentally incapable were being taken care of. Miss Dix had successfully persuaded Congress to pass the "Ten-Million Acre Bill" in 1854. The bill, however, was vetoed by President Franklin Pierce in a veto message which became the hallmark for many decades, upholding "the historic responsibility of the states in matters of social welfare, when people could not sustain their own well-being through self-endeavor or private charity." (Axinn and Levin, 1975, page 37)

The importance of President Pierce's veto of the "Ten-Million Acre Bill" extended far beyond the immediate legislation at hand, for his veto message laid out a philosophical stance that would prevail across many coming decades--in fact, well into the 20th century. Said President Pierce:

> The question presented . . . clearly is upon the constitutionality and propriety of the Federal government assuming to enter into a novel and vast field of legislation, namely that of providing for the care and support of all those among the people of the United States who by any form of calamity become fit objects of public philanthropy. I readily and, I trust, feelingly acknowledge the duty incumbent on us all as men and as among the highest and holiest of our duties, to provide for those who, in the mysterious order of Providence, are subject to want and to disuse of body or mind; but I can not find any authority in the Constitution for making the Federal government the great almoner of public charity throughout the United States. I cannot but believe that it would in the end be prejudicial to the noble offices of charity. . . . If the several States, many of which have already laid the foundation of munificent establishments of local beneficence, and nearly all of which are proceeding to establish them, shall be led to suppose . . . that congress is to make provision for such objects, the fountains of charity will be dried up at home. (President Franklin Pierce, May 3, 1854)

In sum, the residual and institutional orientations represent differing viewpoints of public responsibility for the provision of social welfare services to those in need. The residual formulation looks upon the social welfare system as an emergency network of aid to be used as a temporary source of help until individuals are restored to normal functioning. In contrast, the institutional formulation does not look upon welfare programs as temporary, stopgap mechanisms but as normal functions in a rapidly changing, urban-industrial society. As Heffernan puts it, "Ideologically, a residual conception focuses attention on the failure of the individual in an essentially just society, while the institutional focuses attention on the failure of society to respond to individual needs." (Heffernan, 1979, page 17)

The Three Sectors and Local Human Services

Throughout this text, we shall be dealing with three basic types of systems, or sectors, in our examination of community human services: the governmental, or public sector; the voluntary nonprofit sector; and, the proprietary, or profitmaking sector. These are discussed in more detail in Chapters IV and V below; at this point, we shall only outline the basic character of each one.

The Public Sector

The public sector in the human services is comprised of a series of governmental units at the federal, state, and local levels. In all cases, there are two distinguishing features of public-sector organizations: (1) they are the creations of statutory legislative authority, whether enshrined in constitutional documents or authorized by legislative mandate; and, (2) they are financed directly by tax dollars paid by individuals, business partnerships or corporate businesses.

Public-sector organizations are of three basic types: (1) general-purpose governments, such as federal and state governments, and local municipal, township, and county executive bodies; (2) special-purpose governmental units, such as school districts, that may be independent receivers of tax-dollar funding but are subordinate to local or state general-purpose governments, or both; and (3) agencies of government, which typically are units of general-purpose governments with defined special missions, such as public welfare departments, county children and youth agencies, and the like.

Within the public sector, intergovernmental relations among the various levels--federal, state, and local--and across the different types are important components of the policy, planning, management, and delivery systems for human services. The degree of coordination in these relationships is a critical determinant of the efficiency and effectiveness of community human service systems.

The Voluntary Nonprofit Sector

The voluntary nonprofit sector, sometimes referred to as the "Third Sector" (after government and business), includes a range of not-for-profit, tax-exempt organizations that engage in social welfare, educational, charitable, civic and other functions as part of the overall human services enterprise.

Some voluntary nonprofit organizations carry out their service missions within a defined framework of sectarian values. Others are distinctly not sectarian, supported by corporate and private philanthropic contributions, fees for service, purchase-of-service contracts with public agencies, and third-party reimbursement arrangements with both public and private organizations (e.g., Medicare and Medicaid, Blue Cross, etc.). Most home health agencies, local youth service bureaus, and day care centers fall into this category, as do many community hospitals and senior citizen housing projects.

The voluntary nonprofit sector is sizable. Recent estimates indicate that there were, in 1982, about 132,000 such organizations in the Internal Revenue Service's 501(c)(4) category--primarily social welfare and civic organizations. (Hodgkinson and Weitzman, 1984, page 14)

The Proprietary Sector

This sector consists of human service organizations that are operated for the benefit (profit) of their owners--e.g., individual practitioners, business partners, or corporate shareholders. There are many such organizations in the health services field; for example, proprietary hospitals, nursing homes, and rehabilitation clinics. Proprietary human service providers are increasing in number, especially in areas related to mental health and clinical services.

Chapter IV, which focuses on the range of human service systems in local communities, offers more detail on the different agencies and organizations in the three sectors discussed here. They also form the basis for portions of the discussion found in Chapter V below.

The Concept of Policy

The concept of **policy** is of overarching importance in developing a critical understanding of the planning, management, and delivery of community human services. In this book, we are particularly interested in how policies directed toward human development concerns influence the types of programs and services--both public and private, formal and informal--that exist to meet the human service needs of individuals and groups at the local community level.

Many such policies originate in settings that are remote from the local community. In the case of public-sector policies, federal and state legislative bodies are key actors in the policymaking process. In the private sector, decisionmakers in corporate headquarters are frequently the key actors in formulating policies that are controlling guidelines for the entire corporate system. In both instances, the policies that are formulated serve as authoritative guides to decisions and actions of actors at lower hierarchical levels in the intergovernmental or corporate systems. As such, they act as constraints on the freedom for decisionmaking by those who are subject to the policy stipulations. **Policy space** is a further concept sometimes used to refer to the amount of freedom--or, conversely, the limits of freedom--for decisionmaking allocated to those who are subject to a controlling policy, or set of policies. As we shall see later in this chapter, the "policy space" for local decisionmaking about public human serivces has changed over the past two decades, resulting in a recent "relocalization" of responsibility for human services planning and service delivery. (Gardner, 1976; Agranoff and Robins, 1982)

The concept of **policy** has several different dimensions, all of which are important in understanding the planning and operation of community human service systems. Chapter II provides a detailed

18

exploration of the policy concept and its various dimensions, showing how each relates to human services in local community environments.

Throughout this book, we shall be primarily concerned with **social** policies aimed toward problems and issues in human development and human services. We shall see that human service programs are the products of social policy aims of decisionmakers in both the public and private sectors. Programs, themselves, are the mechanisms for implementing policy goals. Macarov comments that social policies are "deliberate attempts to achieve goals determined by those designated as policymakers. . . . Policies, in turn, are effectuated through . . . programs, which are attempts to carry out the policies (that is, to reach the goals)" (1978, pages 9-10)

It is important to note, however, that social policies--or, for that matter, any form of policy--are not self-implementing. Once formulated and expressed through legislative statutes or executive decrees, policies must be supported by enforcement mechanisms to assure their proper implementation. For example, DeJong and Lifchez (1983) present an interesting policy analysis of the fate of Section 504 of the federal Rehabilitation Act of 1973.

Section 504 specifically bans discrimination against the handicapped in any program or other activity benefiting directly or indirectly from federal financial aid. However, despite the clear intent of Congress regarding the removal of architectural barriers to access to facilities by the handicapped, its enforcement has been carried out with some reluctance by the federal executive branch, especially the Reagan administration, according to DeJong and Lifchez. (1983, page 40) Furthermore, a study conducted by the American Bar Association of state accessibility laws in 1979 indicated that the federal mandate is not implemented with equal forcefulness throughout the nation. (DeJong and Lifchez, 1983, page 46) In effect, the analysis of federal policy toward accessibility of facilities for handicapped individuals clearly demonstrates that any policy simply exists as a **declaration of intent,** unless accompanied by **enforcement and monitoring mechanisms** assuring reasonable implementation of the policy's aims.

The Systems Perspective

The word "system" has become a common part of our everyday vocabulary. Often, we use it in disparaging ways; for example, "the system is wearing me down," or "I can't make heads or tails of the system where I work."

The concept of **system** and the general notion of a "systems perspective" are both important analytical concerns in the human services field. Both enable us to tackle the complex relationships that exist among different levels of social policy formulation and implementation among human service agencies in the same local community, and between these agencies and the clients they attempt to serve. Chapter III of this text is specifically dedicated to an exploration of the systems concept and its application in understanding the different forms of complex relationships that make up the world of the human services.

Van Gigch has commented that every level of life in our modern, complex world confronts us with systems of ideas, organizations, and behaviors that lend some sense of order to what would otherwise be random and chaotic:

> Life in society is organized around complex systems in which, and by which, man tries to bring some semblance of order to his universe. Life is organized around institutions of all sorts: some are man-made, others have developed, it seems, without concerted design. Some institutions, like the family, are small and tractable; others, like politics or industry, are national in scope and becoming more complex every day. Some institutions are privately owned and others belong in the public domain. In every walk of life, whatever our job or our intent, we have to come to grips with organizations and with systems. (Van Gigch, 1974, page 1)

Definitions of the concept of **system** are, for the most part, quite simple in statement. Packard and Fuhriman, for example, offer the following definition: "A system is simply the structure or organization of an orderly whole, clearly showing the interrelations of the parts to each other and to the whole itself." (Packard and

20

Fuhriman, 1973) The related elements can themselves be parts of an organization, such as departments in a public bureaucracy, total organizations, as in the case of interorganizational consortia, or even a theoretical system of related concepts and ideas. The essential ingredient of the concept, however, is the key notion of interrelationships among elements and the ways in which this interrelatedness acts as a mutual influence on the structure or actions of each consituent element of the system.

For example, consider the interrelationships among the among the several systems that play a role in effecting a national public program. (Figure 1.1) The **total** system for the program consists of several different systems that must be linked together for the program to move from conception to implementation. In this instance, what appears in Figure 1.1 as the "constituency systems" consists of voters, taxpaying groups, and other interest groups who influence those who have the final authority for creating the legislation which authorizes the public program; for example, the Congress and the Executive branch of the federal government.

The "authorizing system(s)" component is comprised of those units of the federal government who are recognized by the Constitution as the legitimate decisionmaking bodies for the formulation of national policies and programs. This includes the two houses of Congress and the Executive branch, both of which have specific functions in the legislative and policymaking process.

Once federal legislation becomes law, it must be translated into regulations and guidelines for eventual implementation. This is the function performed by the "administrative systems" of government, usually departments of the executive branch--in the case of human service programs, principally the cabinet departments of Health and Human Services and of Labor.

The next level down in the program system hierarchy consists of the delivery systems, which are responsible for working within the guidelines established by the administrative systems and seeing to it that the services are made available to eligible recipients (or beneficiaries).

The final system level is comprised of the target populations who are the beneficiaries or recipients of the program's services. However, as noted in Figure 1.1, the ability of the hierarchy of interacting systems to "deliver the goods" with respect to the

Figure 1.1

**Systems Involved in the Operation of
a National Public Program**

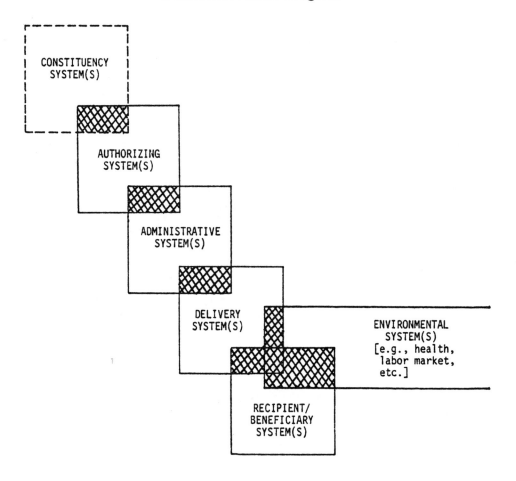

Note: Cross-hatched areas represent important interactions/relationships
between systems.

*Adapted from Leonard Goodwin, "Toward Developing Experimental Social
Research that Constructively Criticizes Public Policies and
Programs," unpublished paper, August 1972.

original policy and program objectives is conditioned by one further system, labeled here the "environmental system(s)." If, for example, the national social program is one aimed towards assuring all elderly citizens of access to health and medical services, such services must themselves be available for this objective to be met. In fact, some sparsely populated rural areas are distinctly lacking in the availability of such services; hence, the "program system" may work but not be supported by the "environmental system." In the same way, a federally sponsored employment and training program may be well designed and the interfaces among the various hierarchical system components functioning smoothly, but if there are no jobs available when training is completed, we again end up with a program whose effectiveness is compromised because of limitations in the program's environmental system(s).

In effect, one purpose of a "systems perspective" in thinking **critically** about human services and human service systems is to avoid the limitations of seeing relationships in simple cause-and-effect terms, thereby overlooking the complexity of intersystem relationships necessary to effect solutions to human development problems. The clinical psychologist who assumes, for example, that the solution to a client's problem can be arrived at without taking into account the individual's systemic relationships with family members, other acquaintances and co-workers, and environmental settings in which the daily activities of life are carried on is engaging in simplistic, linear-causal thinking. As we noted earlier in the citation from Van Gigch, social life "is organized around complex systems," and failure to take account of this complexity is to be extremely myopic, both intellectually and practically. Adopting a systems perspective on the human services--at the policy, planning, management, and service delivery levels--is essential to becoming a competent human development professional.

Social Policy in Action: Job Training Programs

The history of federal, state, and local government involvement in job training programs offers an interesting case example of public social policy and its implementation. A review of

23

governmental support for job training illustrates three things that are fairly typical of public policies and programs for human resource development in the United States.

First, the pattern of federal participation in job training programs exemplifies the oftentimes gradual--some would call it piecemeal--character of the policy process in our federal system. Levitan et al., in their recent review of programs for human resource development in the United States, make the following comment:

> According to dictionary definitions, no policy for human resources now exists. At the federal level most efforts have been a reaction to the special problems--real or imaginary--that caught public attention. Employment and training were funded in a haphazard fashion, in response to perceived needs. (Levitan et al., 1981, page 509)

Morris has also commented that, in the United States, public policy **orientations** toward problems affecting social welfare tend to evolve through a succession of legislative acts. In many instances, the programs brought into being by these legislative actions will gradually add up to a **discernible** policy orientation. However, given the incremental nature of this process, we seldom find, nor should we expect, tidiness in the area of social policy and program development. (Morris, 1979, Chapter 1)

Second, an examination of public-sector job training programs also demonstrates how closely linked social policies and programs are with our system of intergovernmental relationships. The area of job training is not unique in this respect. Rather, it exemplifies how most domestic social programs in the United States are enmeshed in the network of relations among the federal, state, and local levels of government. It also shows how changing philosophies about federal-state-local relationships influence the movement of a program from its point of origin (legislative enactment) to its point of implementation (service delivery).

Third, the history of job training legislation and programs also shows that social policy aims seldom continue unchanged for long periods of time. Changing conditions in the society may warrant new legislation or amendments to existing laws. Social policies are also subject to alteration as public opinion and governmental priorities shift over time.

The Pre-1960 Period

Prior to the onset of the Great Depression of the 1930s, there was little interest within the federal government to regard problems of unemployment or job training as national public issues. The dominant attitude was that any help given to the unemployed should be primarily a state and local responsibility. Only two notable pieces of federal legislation concerned with job training were enacted by Congress in the pre-1930 period, and each dealt with what was perceived as an area of special need.

In 1917, Congress passed the Vocational Education Act. Its purpose was to provide financial support for classroom training of individuals expected to enter the world of work in both agricultural and blue-collar manufacturing jobs. The rationale for this legislation was that, without direct vocational educational training, many of these workers would be "industrially disabled."

In comparison to contemporary levels of federal fiscal support for job training programs, the early Vocational Education Act was a meager effort. It did, however, signal growing recognition of two factors of social change that were invading the world of work: first, that increasing numbers of workers were turning from rural-based agricultural jobs to urban-industrial manufacturing employment, though many were poorly equipped for this change; and second, that new technologies were rapidly changing the character of agricultural production, making the "father-to-son" passing on of knowledge and skills increasingly obsolete in farming.

A second pre-1930 legislative act dealing with job training was the Vocational Rehabilitation Act of 1920. It focused on the training needs of the physically and mentally disabled. Its passage was largely impelled by pressures to provide rehabilitative services to World War I veterans with such disabilities. The act channeled federal funds through state governments to develop and deliver a range of services--for example, prosthetic devices, physical and mental therapy, medical services, and skill training and education--to enhance the employability of the disabled.*

Until the decade of the 1930s, there was very little in the form of a national initiative for involvement of the federal government in employment and job training programs. This only began to change when the enormous unemployment problems of the Great Depression brought these issues into the national spotlight.

As the nation's economic distress deepened in the early 1930s, opposition to federal involvement in programs to aid workers and provide some forms of income security began to diminish, though certainly not disappearing. But unemployment was becoming a **national, public** issue requiring federal intervention of some sort.

One of the earliest legislative actions signaling the federal government's entry into social policies for unemployment problems was the Wagner-Peyser Act of 1933. This legislation established the public employment service, a federal-state partnership program designed to serve workers, employers and the public by providing a national system of employment offices offering counseling, testing, and job placement services without cost to both jobseekers and potential employers.

A second important social program emerging in this period was the unemployment compensation program, which was part of the Social Security Act of 1935. This program assured involuntarily unemployed workers covered by the act of some level of income support while making the transition from one job to another.

A third federal initiative to combat unemployment in the 1930s involved the creation of **temporary** public employment programs. The largest of these, the Works Progress Administration--later named the Works Project Administration--provided federal funds to support jobs for the unemployed in public projects. Others included the National Youth Administration and the Civil Conservation Corps, both aimed toward unemployed youth, with the latter involving rural-based, conservation projects. All of these were

---

*   Both the Vocational Education Act and the Vocational Rehabilitation Act have displayed considerable resiliency. Each has been amended many times. For example, in 1965 the latter was amended to include the "socially disabled"--that is, the economically disadvantaged, or poor--along with its traditional target population of the physically and mentally disabled.

work relief and work training programs and were intended as temporary mechanisms to ameliorate the high rates of unemployment (estimated to be 25% in 1933).

With the coming of World War II, most of the temporary employment programs were disbanded. However, the legislation of the 1930s had clearly established the principle of **federal** responsibility for citizens' welfare. Both the public employment service and the unemployment compensation program became institutionalized as joint federal-state efforts to deal with two important aspects of unemployment problems.

Following World War II, an economic boom and the Korean Conflict of the 1950s resulted in diminished perceptions of a need for new employment or job training legislation. The only notable federal legislation of this period was the Employment Act of 1946. In substance, it was of the variety of legislation referred to by some as "declaratory." (cf. DeJong and Lifchez, 1983) It acknowledged federal responsibility for "maximum employment" but included no provisions for programmatic mechanisms to implement such a lofty aim. The 1946 Act did, however, set up the Council of Economic Advisers (to the President) and the Joint Economic Committee of Congress (serving both House and Senate), and require an annual Economic Report of the President (to the Congress).

It was not until the 1960s that large-scale, federally supported job training and employment programs appeared once again as important parts of the federal legislative agenda. There were several reasons for this new emergence of interest in job training programs. This renewed interest in job training was a product of several growing public concerns, including (1) a fear that automation would create large numbers of "technologically displaced" workers, (2) the increasing number of "pockets of unemployment" created by areas of industrial decline, such as the mining regions of West Virginia, and (3) rising concern about the numbers of poverty-level individuals and households, whose employment and job mobility were restricted by such factors as lack of education and job skills, and racial and language barriers. Consequently, the 1960s witnessed an outpouring of federal legislation aimed towards job training needs as well as other concerns with economic opportunity for low-income populations. This was the decade of the "War on Poverty" and the "Great Society" programs.

In the next parts of this section of the chapter, attention is focused on three major pieces of federal job training legislation in the post-1960 period: the Manpower Development and Training Act of 1962; the Comprehensive Employment and Training Act of 1973; and, the Job Training and Partnershship Act of 1982. Of special interest are differences in the patterns of intergovernmental relationships utilized in each case to implement the social policy goals of job training and employment.

The Manpower Development and Training Act of 1962

The Manpower Development and Training Act (MDTA) of 1962 was the major piece of job training legislation during the 1960s. Its original objective was not directed to the training needs of poorly skilled and low-income populations, but to helping workers **displaced** by automation and technological change. The initial intent of the MDTA was to offering retraining programs to experienced workers, helping them to meet their needs for skills upgrading to keep pace with changing occupational requirements.

In 1963, the Act was amended to provide skills training and education to the unskilled as a means of escaping poverty. Thus, what were generally labeled the "hard-core unemployed" became a primary target for job training services. MDTA programs featured two main types of training: first, institutional training, usually in an established "skills center" training site; and second, on-the-job training with host employers. With the passage of the 1963 amendments, job training programs under the MDTA reflected four basic social policy objectives: (1) to meet labor shortages in specific industries; (2) to provide employment opportunities for the unemployed; (3) to upgrade the labor force, particularly those workers displaced by automation and technological changes in industry; and (4) to provide an escape from poverty.

Job training programs under the MDTA were strongly controlled by agencies of the federal government. The dominant perspective of the time was that superior knowledge and capability for planning and monitoring programs, and allocating resources for their operation throughout all levels of the society resided at the federal level. The relationships established with state and local organizations, both public and private, also reflected what then President Lyndon Johnson characterized as "creative federalism."

As a largely federally planned and controlled effort, funds for MDTA job training programs were awarded to a variety of public and private organizations at the state and local levels. The responsible federal agencies for the various parts of the MDTA dealt directly with these various entities. State and local governments might be involved, but no attempt was made to utilize the intergovernmental system as the principal mechanism for the funding or planning of state or local programs.

The first part of Figure 1.2 depicts the several lines of relationships between the federal government and state and local organizations during the MDTA era. As can be seen, the federal government paid very little attention to the traditional patterns of federal–state–local relationships. In a large number of instances, the line of relationship was direct from the responsible federal agency to local community–based organizations (CBOs), bypassing entirely state or local governments as parties to these relationships.

The Comprehensive Employment and Training Act of 1973

By the end of the 1960s, there was growing concern about the sizable number of employment and training programs spawned by the "Great Society" legislation. There were also growing doubts about the wisdom of excessive control by the federal government of these programs. It was felt that an overabundance of control from Washington often resulted in programs that were "out of touch" and "unresponsive" to local needs. By the beginning of the 1970s, both the public's mood and that of Congress and the Administration were moving toward change.

The Comprehensive Employment and Training Act (CETA) of 1973 resulted in two significant changes in federal policies and programs for job training. First, the act consolidated many of the categorical training programs into a series of special block grants, as a means of reducing fragmentation and overlap. Second, the legislation also emphasized the decentralization of authority and

Figure 1.2
Modal Forms of Intergovernmental Relations in Three
Job Training Programs: MTDA, CETA, and JTPA

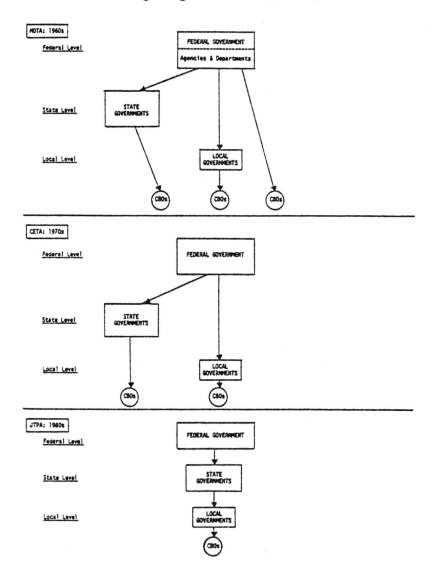

responsibility for program planning and management to state and local government officials. In effect, the "freewheeling" period of federal control was over.

CETA reflected President Nixon's philosophy of a "new federalism," which emphasized the importance of federal–state–local partnerships in the planning and operation of domestic social programs. The Nixon initiative had four basic ingredients: (1) a fundamental reordering of federal–state–local relationships; (2) authority to be placed at the level of government closest to the citizens to be served; (3) primary reliance on local and state government officials for the planning and allocation of training program resources; and (4) federal assistance to be provided in a flexible form, so that local administrators could mount programs tailored to local needs.

The second segment of Figure 1.2 shows the modal pattern of intergovernmental relations as reflected in the implementation of CETA. As can be seen, intergovernmental relationhips were restored to preeminence with respect to policy and program control. It is important to note, though, that President Nixon's version of the "new federalism" did not recognize hierarchical relationships between state and local levels of government. As implemented, the lines of relationship ran directly from the federal to **both** state and local levels, since the majority of "prime sponsors" of local CETA programs were local general-purpose governments or consortia of several local governments in sparsely populated, mostly rural, areas.

The Job Training and Partnership
Act of 1982

The Job Training and Partnership Act (JTPA) was signed into law by President Reagan in 1982, replacing CETA in October of 1983. JTPA continues the policy theme of decentralization of federal control initiated under CETA but strengthens the role of state government in the hierarchy of intergovernmental relations.

The third segment of Figure 1.2 displays the modal pattern of intergovernmental relationships stipulated by JTPA. State governments have a much stronger role under JTPA and are designated as singular conduits for the channeling of federal funds to localities for job training programs. Under JTPA, local areas are organized into "service delivery areas" (SDAs), as approved by the Governor of each state. An SDA may consist of a single local government jurisdiction (a large city or county) or a consortium of several such local general-purpose government jurisdictions, depending on population size.

Another feature of JTPA, setting it apart from its two predecessors, CETA and MDTA, is the prominent role given to local private-sector businesses and industries as equal partners with local government officials in formulating policies and plans for local job training programs. Under JTPA, local "Private Industry Councils" (PICs), which by law must have a majority of private-sector representatives as council members, act as equal partners with local government officials in "signing off" on plans sent to a counterpart State Coordinating Council for approval and funding.

Programmatically, JTPA places very few constraints on local PICs in deciding on priorities and allocations of funds for local job training efforts. Unlike CETA, though, JTPA prohibits the placement of trainees in any type of public-service jobs, even as a transitional employment mechanism. By legislative mandate, funds and training programs are to be targeted toward placement in "unsubsidized jobs"--i.e., only in the private, not the public, sector.

In sum, JTPA modifies the new federalism initiative underlying CETA by adhering closely to the traditional intergovernmental hierarchy of federal to state to local levels of government. Furthermore, it adds to the "relocalization" motif of CETA a theme of "reprivatization" by including private-sector representation as an integral partner with state and local government in the formulation of policies for, as well as the planning and management of, community-based employment and training programs.

A comparative review of MDTA, CETA, and JTPA indicates the importance of understanding prevailing political attitudes regarding intergovernmental relations as a basis for interpreting the organization and management of policymaking and service delivery processes in the human services. Additionally, it underlines the importance of "regime policy" as a dimension of the broader concept of "policy," a topic taken up in detail in Chapter II of this text.

Suggested General Reference Works in Human Services and Social Welfare

This book does not attempt to cover exhaustively the specific types of human services found in local communities. This would not be achievable in an introductory text. There are, however, a number of additional books which a reader might wish to consult to learn more about a particular area of the human services; for example, services to the elderly, home health services, criminal justice, health services, and the like. Below, we have listed several such references.

Anderson, Wayne F., Bernard J. Frieden, and Michael J. Murphy, eds. **Managing Human Services**. Washington, D. C.: International City Management Association, 1977.

Gilbert, Neil, and Harry Specht, eds. **Handbook of the Social Services**. Englewood Cliffs, N. J.: Prentice-Hall, Inc., 1981

Johnson, H. Wayne, ed. **Rural Human Services**. Itasca, Ill.: F. E. Peacock, Publishers, 1980.

Kahn, Alfred J., and Sheila B. Kamerman. **Not for the Poor Alone: European Social Services**. Philadelphia: Temple University Press, 1977.

Kamerman, Sheila B., and Alfred J. Kahn. **Social Services in the United States**. Philadelphia: Temple University Press, 1976.

Mandell, Betty Reid, and Barbara Schram. **Human Services: An Introduction**. New York: John Wiley and Sons, Inc., 1983.

Morris, Robert. **Social Policy of the American Welfare State**. New York: Harper and Row, Publishers, 1979.

National Association of Social Workers. **Encyclopedia of Social Work**. New York: National Association of Social Workers, various editions.

Sauber, S. Richard. **The Human Services Delivery System.** New York: Columbia University Press, 1983.

Schmolling, Paul, R., Merrill Youkeles, and William R. Burger. **Human Services in Contemporary America.** Monterey, Calif.: Brooks/Cole Publishing Company, 1985.

Chapter I

REFERENCES

Agranoff, Robert, ed. **Human Services on a Limited Budget**. Washington, D. C.: International City Management Association, 1983.

Agranoff, Robert, and Alex Pattakos. **Dimensions of Services Integration**. Rockville, Md.: Project SHARE, Human Services Monograph Series, No. 13, 1979.

Agranoff, Robert, and Leonard Robins. "How to Make Block Grants Work: An Intergovernmental Perspective," **New England Journal of Human Services**, 2, Winter 1982, 36-46.

Axinn, June, and Herman Levin, eds. **Social Welfare: A History of the American Response to Need**. New York: Dodd, Mead & Company, 1975.

Brace, Charles Loring. **The Dangerous Classes in New York**. New York: Wynkoop and Hallenbeck, 1880.

Buell, Bradley et al. **Community Planning for Human Services**. New York: Columbia University Press, 1952.

DeJong, Gerben, and Raymond Lifchez. "Physical Disability and Public Policy," **Scientific American**, 248, June 1983, 40-49.

Dobelstein, Andrew H. **Politics, Economics, and Public Welfare**. Englewood Cliffs, N. J.: Prentice-Hall, Inc., 1980

Gardner, Sidney. **Roles for General Purpose Governments in Services Integration**. Rockville, Md.: Project SHARE, Human Services Monograph Series, No. 2, 1976.

Gilbert, Neil. "The Transformation of Social Services," **Social Services Review**, 51, December, 1977, 624-641.

Goodwin, Leonard. "Toward Developing Experimental Social Research That Constructively Criticizes Public Policies and Programs." Unpublished paper, August 1972.

Heffernan, W. Joseph. **Introduction to Social Welfare Policy: Power, Scarcity and Common Human Needs**. Itasca, Ill.: F. E. Peacock, Publishers, Inc., 1979.

Hodgkinson, Virginia Ann, and Murray S. Weitzman. **Dimensions of the Independent Sector: A Statistical Profile**. Washington, D. C.: Independent Sector, 1984.

Huttman, Elizabeth D. **Introduction to Social Policy**. New York: McGraw Hill Publishing Co., Inc., 1981.

Kramer, Ralph M. "From Voluntarism to Vendorism," in **Public-Private Collaboration in the Delivery of Local Public Services**. Davis, Calif.: University of California-Davis, Institute of Governmental Affairs, 1980, pp. 62-74.

Levitan, Sar A., Garth L. Mangum, and Ray Marshall. **Human Resources and Labor Markets**, 3rd ed. New York: Harper and Row, Publishers, 1981.

Macarov, David. **The Design of Social Welfare**. New York: Holt, Rinehart, and Winston, 1978.

35

Macarov, David. **Work and Welfare: The Unholy Alliance.** Beverly Hills, Calif.: Sage Publicatons, Inc., 1980.

Magill, Robert S. **Community Decision Making for Social Welfare.** New York: Human Sciences Press, 1979.

Mandell, Betty Reid, and Barbara Schram. **Human Services: An Introduction.** New York: John Wiley and Sons, Inc., 1983.

Mills, C. Wright. **The Sociological Imagination.** New York: Oxford University Press, 1959.

Morris, Robert. **Social Policy of the American Welfare State.** New York: Harper and Row, Publishers, 1979.

Morris, Robert. "The Human Services Function in Local Government," in **Managing Human Services**, ed. Wayne F. Anderson, Bernard J. Frieden, and Michael J. Murphy. Washington, D. C.: International City Management Association, 1977, pp. 5-36

Naisbitt, John. **Megatrends.** New York: Warner Books, Inc., 1982.

Packard, T., and A. Fuhriman. "Basic Concepts of Systems analysis," **Journal of Employment Counseling,** 10, 1973, 100-107

Peirce, Neal R. "New Federalism and the Social Services: Friend or Foes?" **New England Journal of Human Services,** 2, Summer 1982, 13-19.

Pierce, President Franklin. **Veto Message to Congress, May 3, 1854.**

Pumphrey, Ralph E. "Compassion and Protection: Dual Motivations in Social Welfare," **Social Services Review,** 33, March 1959, 21-29.

Romanyshyn, John. **Social Welfare: From Charity to Justice.** New York: Random House, 1971.

Rutter, Laurence. **The Essential Community: Local Government in the Year 2000.** Washington, D. C.: International City Management Association, 1980.

Sauber, S. Richard. **The Human Services Delivery System.** New York: Columbia University Press, 1983.

Warren, Roland L., ed. **New Perspectives on the American Community.** 3rd ed. Chicago: Rand McNally Publishing Company, 1977.

Wilensky, Harold L., and Charles N. Lebeaux. **Industrial Society and Social Welfare.** New York: Russell Sage Foundation, 1958.

Zald, Mayer "Demographics, Politics, and the Future of the Welfare State," **Social Services Review,** 51, May 1977, 110-124.

Chapter II

THE POLICY CONCEPT: BASIC DIMENSIONS

"Kings will be tyrants from policy, when
subjects are rebels from principle."
–Edmund Burke

Introduction

Policies permeate and regulate our lives. Much more than we realize, the actions of decision makers who are often remote from us in distance (and even in time) influence our well-being and channel our daily actions. We generally associate the concept of "policy" with governments and other large institutions, such as business corporations, labor unions, professional associations, universities, and other formal organizations. Without question, many aspects of our total society and the various environments we encounter daily are affected by the policies of such organizations.

Each of us, however, is also involved with policy in much more direct and intimate ways. Individuals also formulate, advocate and pursue specific policies as guides to their own actions and to their relationships with others. In short, we all make and implement policies every day.

Our consideration of the policy concept begins at this "personal policy" level. After "getting into policy thinking" on the personal level, we shall move on to examine a number of definitions of the concept offered by specialists in the field of policy analysis. This is followed by what is essentially the core of the chapter; namely, a general typology of policies and an examination of the relationship of fundamental social values to sectoral public policy, regime policy, jurisdictional policy, administrative policy, and street-level policy. In all instances, of course, our ultimate concern is focused on human services and their implementation in local community environments. Throughout the chapter, you will become increasingly aware of the importance of policies as the principles and goals that facilitate and constrain the operation of community and human services.

An Exercise In Personal Policy

Think, for a moment, about a piece of equipment or an appliance that you own: for example, a stereo, a camera, a bicycle, or an automobile. Do you allow other people to use it? To borrow it? Would you loan it to a friend? A stranger? Your parents? A college professor? A seven-year-old girl or boy? A mentally retarded person? How about an E.T.? An escaped convict? A person with a severe heart problem? After pondering these questions, complete the following sentences.

I would consider loaning my _____(item)

to a _____, _____, _____, and _____.

I would not loan it to _____, _____, _____, or _____.

Now, list the criteria you used to decide the types of people who would be eligible potential borrowers of your equipment or appliance. Some examples of these criteria might be the value of the item, the closeness (or remoteness) of each borrower's relationship to you, their qualifications to operate the item, their experience and training, their "need" for it, and the nature of intended use. List your criteria below.

Criterion A: _____
Criterion B: _____
Criterion C: _____
Criterion D: _____
Criterion X: _____

(If you feel that you would not loan this item "under any condition," state this and list your reasons for your decision.)

Chapter I introduced you to the idea of "policy space" as an important consideration in making decisions about policies and programs in the human services. As a useful concept in the study of policy decisions, it refers to the range within which limits may be placed on decisions about a policy and its implementation. In thinking about your "personal policy" illustration, consider any conditions you would place on the loan of your equipment or appliance. For example, may it be used only for a certain period of time? In a certain geographical area? Under certain weather conditions? Is it available for certain uses but not for others? A party? An essential function? For pleasure? For work?

Now, list your conditions for making the loan and, after that, list any instructions for use, maintenance, repair or damage.

Conditions for loan:

Condition 1: _____
Condition 2: _____
Condition 3: _____
Condition n: _____

Instructions for use, maintenance, repair, etc.

Instr. a: _____
Instr. b: _____
Instr. c: _____
Instr. x: _____

Finally, consider the following questions. What principles guided your policy on loaning the item? What is your **general** perspective on loaning things to others? (For example, one option might be your feeling that "people ought to take care of their own needs, and I keep things for myself." Or, you might feel that "loaning and borrowing are means for mutual benefit, ways of helping others and getting help occasionally.") You should also consider what values you applied in arriving at your general perspective on loaning. For example, any of the following could be a statement of an underlying value premise for your personal policy. "One ought to share with a friend, relative, or close acquaintance." "It's unwise to let just anyone use your equipment." (Why?) "I like to try to help someone in need." "Let them take care of their own problems." "Someone must really show a need, and that she or he is a responsible person."

Think about it for a moment, and then list the values that you believe support your policy.

Value 1: _____
Value 2: _____
Value 3: _____
Value 4: _____
Value n: _____

If you've completed this exercise, you have articulated a personal policy statement. In fact, it may be a fairly complex policy, including eligibility criteria, principles for conditional use, and requirements for use. Additionally, you have declared a number of basic values on which the policy is based.

Each of us makes many decisions each day which are based on such "personal policies," regardless of how conscious we may be about the "policy process" in our personal lives. We typically do this without much consideration of either the values or the general principles which support our decisions, or the criteria they impose. Realization of this fact now makes it possible for you to consider the nature of policy and to begin to make explicit decisions and plans. Think for a moment about your personal "policy" in other areas. What is your policy about blind dates? On studying? On attending classes regularly? What is your position on recreation? On jogging? On sex? The fact is that personal policies permeate your life, just as policies permeate the social programs of public and private agencies, and the corporate lives of private businesses. Policies provide guides to evaluating potential actions and behavior; actions, in turn, reflect policies that have been formally established (explicit policies) or have come about through tradition or habitual usage (implicit policies). Now, let's consider some of the formal definitions of "policy" presented in the literature.

What Is A Policy?

The word "policy" is derived from the Greek words **politeia** and **polis** which refer to the "state" and "citizenship," and the Latin **politia,** which literally means the "administration of the commonwealth." Thus, at its base, policy refers to the regulation of morals, safety, social order and welfare of a "body politic"--whether this be an organization, a community, state or nation.

The use of the term today, however, particularly in reference to community and human service systems, takes on additional dimensions and applications. Contemporary usage accepts a wide range of decisions and actions which guide or regulate behavior as reflecting "policy": for example, "corporate policy," "agency policy," "union policy," "church policy," and "personal policy," to name a few. (The next chapter, on "systems," will provide a basis for making finer distinctions among policy-making units and their role in community human services systems.) In addition, the concept may be used to designate intended or actual actions, decisions, or the policymaking process itself. Rather than adopt a rigid set of definitions for policy, any one of which would be inadequate for understanding the variety which exists in the field, we shall consider several definitions. (This approach of "tuning into the field" will be used throughout the book.) Consider the following definitions.

> **. . . a web of decisions and actions that allocates values.**
> —David Easton

41

Actual and potential government [or private] programs and actions designed to cope with various social problems.

-Policy Studies Organization

AT ITS CORE, POLICY IS A COURSE OF ACTION INTENDED TO ACCOMPLISH SOME END.

-H. Hugh Heclo

A guide to action in future unanticipated situations. Policy identifies the general principles which an individual party or a government uses to make choices and decisions in unfamiliar circumstances which may arise in the future.

-Robert Morris

A set of interrelated decisions taken by a political actor or group of actors concerning the selection of goals and the means of achieving them within a specified situation where these decisions would, in principle, be within the power of these actors to achieve.

-W. I. Jenkins

In whatever loci it occurs, policy is above all, strategies, actions, or plans for alleviating a social problem or meeting a social need after analyzing alternative choices.

-David Gil

A purposive course of action followed by an actor or set of actors in dealing with a problem or matter of concern.

-James Anderson

PRINCIPLES WHICH GUIDE PRESENT AND FUTURE DECISIONS.

-Hyman and Miller

Policies result from the decisions of actors to think and behave in certain ways. They make explicit the principles, goals or patterns of actions of an actor (or set of actors) regarding a particular issue or problem. Policies make regular what otherwise would be random, chaotic or arbitrary decisionmaking or actions. As premises for decisionmaking, policies provide guidance, direction and a degree of predictability to the behavior of individuals, groups and organizations.

Some Examples Of Policies

Policies may be quite vague or very specific in their terms of reference. For example, it was not long ago that social caseworkers had considerable discretion under existing public welfare policies to decide whether a poor person was "truly needy" and "worthy" before providing financial aid. Today, as a result of court decisions and subsequent legislative acts, there are strict criteria to determine eligibility, based on income, assets, and availability for work.

Policies may also be as elusive and intangible as a vague intention or general plan to "do something" about a problem. Or, they may be highly explicit, specifying in detail the goals and principles which guide decisions and actions. In fact, a policy may involve an actual decision or rule to guide or control behavior, such as a statutory law or regulation. Or, policy may sometimes refer to the action itself, or a series of more-or-less related actions of a person, organization, or government.

Consider the following examples of policies. As you do so, attempt to identify the responsible actor, organization or authority.

o **A comprehensive final examination (or final paper in lieu of an examination) is required for all courses at The Pennsylvania State University.**

o **Because the federal government considers them as "not available for work," as required by law, college students are generally not eligible for food stamps.**

o   The State of Pennsylvania has legislation containing financial incentives to encourage local communities to establish and support hospice programs for the terminally ill.

o   In the United States, professional nurses may choose not to implement a physician's orders if they disagree with them but cannot alter a physician's prescribed medications, even though they might have the knowledge and training to do so.

o   In some states, a driver under the influence of alcohol who is involved in an accident which kills another person is guilty of manslaughter--even though the accident may have been the fault of another person.

o   A university's policy on academic dishonesty indicates that copying the work of others or looking at the exams of others during a test are punishable offenses which may lead to expulsion from the class and an automatic grade of "F."

o   An unemployed person in the United States with an established work record may receive unemployment compensation, while a recently widowed housewife of 20 years with two pre-school children who is also unemployed but has never worked for wages outside the household may not.

o   A city council authorizes the use of funds and the local police department's services in helping neighborhood groups to form "crime watch" programs for different areas of the city.

o   An amendment to the federal Social Security Act increases the amount elderly citizens must pay out

of their own pockets in order to qualify for Medicare benefits.

It is clear from these brief examples that policies have a ubiquitous influence on human affairs, extending through all levels of social organization and pervading all types of human service issues and problems. How, then, to get a "handle" on the concept and use it as a tool in understanding programs and planning in the area of human development? To do this, we shall use a typology of policies to provide some order amidst this complexity. The typology begins with the most general, almost intangible, level of "policy" and gradually narrows down to more specific levels of laws, regulations and actions.

A Typology Of Social Policies

From the outset, we should make it clear that our main interest in this section and the remainder of the chapter is on **social** policy as a principal concern in understanding community systems and human services. The following general definition of social policy, offered by Huttman, provides a foundation for our subsequent consideration of a typology of social policies relevant to human development concerns.

> The aims of social policy measures are to assist people in need of help to alleviate social problems, to improve the individual's and the group's social and economic situation, and to provide an environment conducive to growth and satisfaction . . . . Social policies, as plans of action and strategies for providing services, also have the goal of improving intrasocial human relations by eliminating the dysfunctioning of individuals and groups caused by external forces and personal problems. In sum, the policymaker's overall goal is to improve the quality of life and circumstances of living of individuals and groups. (Huttman, 1981, p. 5)

Morris (1979, p.16) sets out a typology for social policy analysis which provides a framework for distinguishing among several "levels" of types of policy. We have adapted this system of classification in order to provide some order to our concerns in considering different forms of social policy. The six categories of policy are the following:

Societal Policy: The social values and aspirations, principles, customs and institutions which form the fundamental criteria for evaluating worth, rightness and justice in a society. In discussing this particular category of social policy, Morris notes that the social norms underlying societal policy "determine what a society will allow its organized structure of governance to do on behalf of its members."

Regime Policy: The principles which a particular set of ruling authorities use in approaching the task of decisionmaking and governing.

Sectoral Public Policy or Community Subsystem Policy: The guiding principles for decisionmaking and action used by a government or other organizations in defining and responding to perceived needs, goals and problems of its citizens or members. Subsystem policies address specific aspects of community life; for example, health, housing, justice, welfare, and the like.

Jurisdictional Policy and Laws: The general principles and laws of specific jurisdictional authorities: federal, state and local governments; private and voluntary organizations.

Administrative Policy and Regulations: The rules and regulations promulgated by public or private organizations to implement the above, and to make explicit the expected behavior of organizational personnel.

Delivery-Level, or Street-Level, Policy and Procedure:
The behavior and/or principles adopted by individuals in carrying out administrative policies and regulations. These may conform to, be more restrictive than, or expand upon the principles of the foregoing, higher levels of policy.

These general categories allow us to differentiate among types and levels of policy in any governmental unit, organization, or community. It should also be kept in mind that there are distinctions between policies (of all types) which reflect **intentions** or **plans** as guides for formulating action, and policies which are manifest in **actions** or a **series of related actions** based on underlying policy principles. The following subsections explicate each of these types or levels of policy, showing how they apply in understanding contemporary American communities and human services systems.

Societal Policy: Social Values And Aspirations

The most general level of rules and principles which guide policy involves the values and normative standards of a group or an entire society. While many observers may not consider such cultural values as "policy" per se, it is clear that society and group norms often provide fundamental guides and criteria for decisionmaking and action in the policy realm. Max Weber, a social scientist of the late 19th and early 20th centuries who laid much of the groundwork for contemporary sociology and organizational theory, noted the following about social policy:

> The distinctive characteristic of social policy is indeed the fact that it cannot be resolved merely on the basis of purely technical considerations which assume already settled ends. Normative standards of value can and must be the objectives of dispute in discussion of a problem in social policy because the problem lies in the domain of general cultural values. (Weber, 1949)

According to Morris, societal policy, as expressed in cultural norms and aspirations, "means the premises, values, and general mind-set of the country. Such values shape our political choices, and our scientific and technological pathways for exploration." (1979, p. 17) Some of the dominant norms which undergird the other levels of social policy in the United States include (1) a belief in the efficacy of a capitalist, market-oriented economy, (2) the correctness of democratic decisionmaking as a basic framework for resolving disputes over policy options, (3) pursuit of "success" and well-being through diligence and hard work, (4) individual responsibility for self and family, except in unusual or emergency conditions, (5) a belief in technology and economic progress as the answer to social problems and inequities, (6) security of the individual from unreasonable government intervention, and (7) equal rights for all classes of citizens.

While these normative principles may be said to reflect **dominant** values and norms in American society, they do not exist without challenge. Social policies, and the normative standards which underlie them, are the outcome of social disagreements and conflicts about justice, equity, and the ordering of affairs in the communities where citizens reside. Thus, the emergence and formalization of social policies are frequently attended by opposition, and the existence of disagreement leads to continuing evolution of ideas and/or conflict over the proper ends of such policies. Consider, for example, the following statements of prominent Americans, some past and some present, which are reflective of some of the basic values in the United States. As you consider these sections, note too that there exists a good deal of disagreement about the basic values and normative standards, and that gradual evolution tends to occur over time.

>>To what extent do you and people you know have elements of these sentiments in your personal value systems? Are the different perspectives present? Most of us have elements of each of these values in our personality subsystem. We use them in personal policymaking and

decisions. Often, they create dissonances and conflicts within as we ponder which ones to apply to specific situations. So, too, for the broader community system and subsystems--but at a greater degree of complexity.<<

Capitalism and Success

Traditional societies are characterized by repetition of cultural patterns from generation to generation. The United States, as a modern industrialized nation, however, has been characterized by a belief in change, and that change is best accomplished through **individual initiative** and hard work expressed through a **capitalist economic system.** In "The Art of Money Getting," P. T. Barnum put it this way:

> In the United States, where we have more land than people, it is not at all difficult for persons in good health to make money. In this comparatively new field there are so many avenues of success open, so many vocations which are not crowded, that any person of either sex who is willing, at least for the time being, to engage in any respectable occupation that offers, may find lucrative employment. (Barnum, 1879)

Henry David Thoreau, in "Life Without Principle," however, paints a word picture of a parallel longing of many Americans--the desire for "the good life" as manifest in leisure.

> . . . Let us consider the way in which we spend our lives. This world is a place of business. What an infinite bustle! I am awaked almost every night by the panting of the locomotive. It interrupts my dreams. There is no sabbath. It would be glorious to see mankind at leisure for once. It is nothing but work, work, work. (Thoreau, 1906)

While the predominant value would suggest that the "measure of a man" is his or her ability to make money, there is a significant proportion of the population which finds satisfaction in other pursuits. Thus, a conflict tends to exist over this basic value, which in turn is manifest in disputes over policies and programs.

Diligence and Hard Work

If success is measured by making money through the capitalist system of free enterprise, other dominant values stress that satisfaction and well-being are achieved by working at productive occupations. Max Weber pointed out the importance of this "protestant work ethic" to industrialization, calling it the "spirit of capitalism." However, American society has always had an independently wealthy elite that did not "work" in the usual sense, and today's "jet setters" provide additional models for a new wealthy elite. There is also a recognition in contemporary society that structural unemployment is a continuing fact of life for a significant proportion of the population and that many jobs do not provide the soul-satisfying employment promised by dominant values. Booker T. Washington and Paul Goodman provide contrasting illustrations of these perspectives:

> Our harvest is always in proportion to the amount of earnest labour that we put into our work. A farmer who puts earnest effort into his field work will reap a profitable harvest. The student who puts earnest effort into a lesson will get pleasure and satisfaction from it. . . . In either case, when he has performed his duty, his conscience will be clear; he will be free from any restraint; he will have courage to face the obligations which confront all of us in the battle of life. . . . In every pursuit of life, it may be accepted as an axiom that we get out of every effort just what we put into it of hard, honest labour. (Washington, 1900)

It's hard to grow up when there isn't enough man's work. There is "nearly full employment" (with highly significant exceptions), but there get to be fewer jobs that are necessary or unquestionably useful; that require energy and draw on some of one's best capacities; and that can be done keeping one's honor and dignity.

. . .

It is hard for the young man now to maintain his feelings of justification, sociability, and serviceability. (Goodman, 1960)

While there is a growing recognition in American societal policy that social conditions beyond the control of specific individuals are responsible for much dependence, the underlying policy values stress providing for oneself and one's family through work. These dominant values consider the poor to be so because of conditions under their control--if they would just get a job and manage their money better, they would not have such problems.

The gospel of wealth inevitably implied a philosophy of poverty. Poverty should be for the individual a temporary status. With initiative, industry, and ability he should rise above it. For the masses who do not rise, poverty must be a badge of failure proclaiming that the individual is defective in capacity or morals or both. The philosophy emphasized individual responsibility. It implied that the democratic doctrine of the free individual has no meaning, if the individual citizen is not willing to buy his liberty at the price of responsibility.

The gospel of wealth assumed that the poor, the less fortunate in the competition of the market, would accept the leadership of the men who [rose] to the top. (Gabriel, 1956, p. 169)

Community Aid for the Weak and Helpless

While individuals are generally expected to take care of themselves and their families through hard work and income earned in the marketplace of capitalist enterprise, these principles have been tempered by a social concern for those who cannot help themselves. The Judeo-Christian ethic is no doubt the root of our values regarding the virtues of charity: there is a community responsibility to be "My Brother's Keeper." One manifestation of the ancient Hebrew laws requiring care for the widowed and helpless is a belief in aid to the weak and helpless, and community aid to others in times of trouble. This perspective views the individual acquisitiveness of capitalism as ultimately selfish and greedy. The principles of love and charity set forth in the Sermon on the Mount articulate a severe guide to societal responsibility for others: "Do Unto Others As You Would Have Them Do Unto You." Specific responsibilities are related in the parable of the last judgment:

> When the Son of man comes . . . he will separate [all the nations] one from another as a shepherd separates the sheep from the goats. . . . Then the King will say to those on his right hand, 'Come, O blessed of my Father, inherit the kingdom prepared for you from the foundation of the world; for I was hungry and you gave me food, I was thirsty and you gave me drink, I was naked and you clothed me, I was sick and you visited me, I was in prison and you came to me.' Then the righteous will answer him, 'Lord, when did we see thee hungry and feed thee, or thirsty and give thee drink? And when did we see thee a stranger and welcome thee, or naked and clothe thee? And when did we see thee sick or in prison and visit thee?' And the King will answer them, 'Truly, I say to you, as you did it to one of the least of these my brethren, you did it to me.' (Matthew 25: 31-39)

Thus, there is a strong belief that the broader community should be responsible for vulnerable individuals and groups. As noted by Morris:

> The accepted definition of vulnerable individuals is limited mainly to certain groups who are perceived to be relatively weak and helpless--the aged, widows, orphans, the crippled, and by recent extension, anyone in serious trouble not of his or her own making, as, for example, unemployment following an acceptable work history. (Morris, p. 20)

Such community responsibility has traditionally favored neighborliness and service by religious charities to help people in such straits. The decline of community as sharing of responsibility among a relatively small group of people on a first-name basis, however, led to the need for more organized approaches. Thus, we had the emergence of a sizable health and welfare effort by private, voluntary organizations; and then when this proved to be inadequate to bear the full responsibility, various levels of government aid were initiated. The development of social security, which was initiated during the depression of the 1930s, and the "War on Poverty" of the 1960s are major manifestations of such "community aid" values.

Government involvement with the weak and helpless has typically been seen as a "last resort" option, and the growing involvement of the public sector in the human services in recent decades has now come under attack. We shall see in a later chapter that these "Brother's Keeper" principles have gradually broadened to include more groups and a wider part of the spectrum of human need; and the concept of minimum aid in emergencies has been challenged by the concept that an adequate standard of living should be assured for all citizens as a fundamental right.

Technology and Progress

Belief in continual progress through the development of new technology has been a precept of American thought since Revolutionary times. The nation was founded by people who were determined to be masters of their own destiny, and it was populated by successive waves of immigrants pursuing a new life. Principles of individualism and capitalism were accompanied by a belief in the perfectibility of Man and the Society in which he lives. American invention and ingenuity had an essential role to play in transforming a rude, nasty, brutish life into one of civilized order and contentment. The cotton gin, the steam engine, the telegraph and telephone, the automobile and the electric light were but precursors of home computers, microwave ovens, and space travel. As geographic frontiers were conquered, technological frontiers remained. In 1900 Charles Sumner observed:

> Wherever we turn is progress--in science, in literature, in knowledge of the earth, in knowledge of the skies, in intercourse among men, in the spread of liberty, in the works of beneficence, in the recognition of Human Brotherhood. . . . Men everywhere, breaking away from the past, are pressing on to the things that are before.
>
> . . .
>
> Let me state the law [of human progress] as I understand it. Man, as an individual, is capable of indefinite improvement. Societies and nations . . . are capable of indefinite improvement. And this is the destiny of man, of societies, of nations, and of the Human Family. (Sumner, 1900)

The industrial revolution had not run its course, however, when some people began to realize that America's natural resources were not endless. The practice of uncontrolled exploitation of natural resources to promote Man's material wealth was challenged by those who saw the shale pits and culm banks of the Northeast, and the dust bowls and ravaged forests of the West. Values stressing the conservation of natural resources were manifest most dramatically in the Presidency of Theodore Roosevelt (1901-1909). The conservation ethic now tempers principles of capitalist exploitation with a concern for the land and the future.

> The old rapists--the lumbermen and miners and utility companies--are still with us, though today they substitute seduction for rape wherever possible. The Georgia-Pacific Company still strips virgin Douglas fir from California's northern coast, but today it also contributes a few thousand dollars to a study of the habits and habitats of the American eagle.

. . .

> But . . . new rapists are loose upon the land. . . . They
> are called Engineers. They build bridges and dams and
> highways and causeways and flood control projects. They
> **manage** things. They commit rape with bulldozers.
> (Marine, 1967)

A corollary to these values is a belief in **education for the masses** as essential to the good life. Education prepares people to understand and to use technology intelligently; and it creates new waves of scientists to push back the frontiers of science in the interest of all. Thus, there is a belief that today's problems will be resolved by technological innovation in the long run. In fact, the two strains in this value set, illustrated above, come together at times to lead to a belief that even the problems of hunger, poverty, pollution, land use, housing, and depletion of natural resources can be resolved through technological innovation.

Democratic Process and Security of the Person Against Arbitrary Governmental Control

> We hold these truths to be self-evident, that all
> men are created equal, that they are endowed by their
> creator with certain unalienable Rights, that among those
> are Life, Liberty, and the Pursuit of Happiness. That to
> secure these rights, Governments are instituted among
> Men, deriving their just powers from the consent of the
> governed. That whenever any form of Government
> becomes destructive of these ends, it is the Right of the
> people to alter or abolish it, and to institute new
> Government, laying its foundation on such principles and
> organizing its powers in such form, as to them shall seem
> most likely to effect Safety and Happiness. (Declaration
> of Independence, 1776)

The right to participate in government and the right to be free from unreasonable and arbitrary governmental control are inextricably intertwined in the values of Americans. While forceful revolution was necessary because of a despotic government, the democratic process provides a means for continuing change. Reform through participation in the governing process is the American ideal. Fundamental to American values is the principle that as long as free people of good will cooperate in the democratic process, order, individual rights, and progressive change can be assured.

> If you accept a democratic system, this means that you are prepared to put up with those of its workings, legislative or administrative, with which you do not agree as well as with those that meet with your concurrence. This willingness to accept, in principle, the workings of a system based on the will of the majority, even when you yourself are in a minority, is simply the essence of democracy. Without it there could be no system of representative self government at all. (Kennan, 1968)

The **democratic consent of the governed** is thus an essential ingredient of the American system of government. The Revolution, and the conditions which created it, however, raised the specter of tyranny and domination. Thus, the framers of the Constitution created a system of checks and balances to avoid undue control by any individual or group. An elaborate set of rights of individuals, which the government is responsible for assuring, is designed to elaborate the principles of, and to place constraints on, government actions:

> "Freedom can exist only where the citizen is assured that his person is secure against bondage, lawless violence, and arbitrary arrest and punishment." (The Presidential Commission on Civil Rights, 1947)

> "The history of American freedom is, in no small measure, the history of procedure." (Justice Frankfurter)

Ingrained in American values are certain "rights" which are deemed necessary to informed and free participation in government. Among them are the rights of free speech, of peaceful assembly, the right of the governed to vote for their governors, and to petition the government for redress of grievances. Thus, the option to participate in the power process is a key value in the American system.

Freedom from **unreasonable government intervention** is valued both as essential to individualism, and as a control on threats to political opposition. Thus, rights **against** unreasonable searches and seizures, blanket or unspecific search warrants, arbitrary arrest and punishment, self-incrimination and double jeopardy are firmly ingrained in American values, laws and procedures. Similarly, the right to counsel, public trial by jury, fair and speedy trials, and bail are also bulwarks against government suppression of individuals.

For over two hundred years, the American system has tried to reconcile these values of participation and freedom from government interference, with the need for governmental control to maintain order and to protect individuals from the harmful acts of others. The federal system restricts the central government to only those powers explicitly delegated to it. Remaining powers rest with the states and local governments which are closer to the direct control of the citizenry and fragmented into fifty separate state systems. Americans thus sacrifice efficiency in decisionmaking and uniformity of laws to diversity and protection of the individual.

Equal Rights for all Americans

All persons born or naturalized in the United States, and subject to the jurisdiction thereof, are citizens of the United States and of the State wherein they reside. No State shall make or enforce any law which shall abridge the privileges or immunities of citizens of the United States; nor shall any State deprive any person of life, liberty, or property without due process of law, nor deny to any person within its jurisdiction the equal protection of the laws. (U.S. Constitution Fifteenth Amendment, July 28, 1868)

The right of citizens of the United States to vote shall not be denied or abridged by the United States or by any State on account of sex. (U.S. Constitution, Nineteenth Amendment, August 18, 1920)

Fundamental to the exercise of the basic values of Americans is the principle of equal protection under the law. The most basic documents on which this country was founded assert the belief that "All Men Are Created Equal." The achievement of these rights for all groups, however, is an area where change has occurred continually, but sporadically.

Racial and ethnic minorities have frequently been treated as less than equal, and even the original Constitution defined a black person as two-thirds of a man for voting purposes. As the Civil War was being fought , the Irish were rioting in the Northeast in protest againt ethnic discrimination. Other groups, too, have suffered as the objects of narrow-mindedness and bigotry: Chinese, Japanese, Korean and other Asian groups, as well as Germans, Swedes, Italians, Poles and other Eastern European groups, have been the objects of ridicule and discrimination in the past, and efforts continue to assure equal rights, even as the nation is host to new immigrants from Latin America, Southeast Asia, and other parts of the world. (Recall also that women were considered to be represented by their husbands in the voting booth until the Nineteenth Amendment was passed in 1920. And in 1984, Mississippi became one of the last states to ratify this amendment.)

The Civil War, the equal rights amendments to the Constitution and Supreme Court decisions of over a century were precursors to the Civil Rights Movement of the 1950s and 1960s. Rallies, mass demonstrations, civil disobedience and violence accompanied the movement, whose supporters demanded their constitutional rights in education, housing, employment, social services, police protection, and voting. The Civil Rights Act of 1964, several major court decisions, comparable laws in states and local governments and the continuing efforts of millions of Americans translated these efforts into more specific levels of policy.

Equal rights continues to be supported as a national goal, but its implementation is imperfect and inadequate in many areas. "Affirmative action" for racial, ethnic and sexual minorities is alternately supported as a means to repair past damages, and opposed as "reverse discrimination." At the same time there are those who advocate expanding equal rights principles to additional groups such as cultists, homosexuals, the unborn and other identifiable categories. The resolution of the conflict between equal rights and individual liberty is a fundamental source of tension and change in the American system.

Values As Policies

Social values provide the most fundamental level of principles and guides for societal decisions and actions. They put severe boundaries around what a people will tolerate. This "political culture" varies from society to society and to a degree, from group to group within a society. The United States operates within a generally capitalist economic system and a democratic political system. Suggestions of fundamental change of the economy to a fascist corporate state or to a collectivist socialist state are almost universally opposed (although there are groups that would support each). Many other political cultures, however, have non-capitalist economic values. Success through making money and hard work may be important in the U.S. and other Western industrialized countries; success through emulating one's forefathers and making do with what life offers is prevalent in some other nations. Community aid for the weak and helpless runs through the American political culture. In some countries community aid for everyone is expected; and in still others, it is "every man for himself."

American federalist democratic ideals of equal participation and protection from government abuses are not shared universally. Most countries have some form of authoritarian rule with centralist control. One is guilty until proven innocent. Detention of citizens in prision for political reasons is frequent.

Clearly, political culture is unique for each nation. It puts fundamental limits on which policies are most likely to be adopted. We shall see that these principles apply to nations as polities, **and** for subsystems such as states, counties, corporations, specific programs, groups and other types of "community." (In fact, nations can be considered as subsystems of the international community.) The next chapter on systems and subsystems will examine this latter issue in more detail. First, let us examine the remaining categories of policy.

Regime Policy

The second type of policy we shall consider reflects the principles applied by a governing administration or current set of authorities. The American democratic system provides for periodic replacement of governmental authorities. Different political parties, each with a different political "platform" or sets of policies, vie for the support of the public in electoral forums. Comparable alternating or changing of leaders also occurs in private business and industrial organizations and in voluntary nonprofit organizations. "Regime policy" refers to the principles which underlie a particular direction or emphasis for policy as espoused by an incumbent set of leaders; it thus tends to be less general and more time-limited than societal values and norms.

Clearly, regime policies pose potential directions for policy, and often a substantial change in policy directions. For example, the "Great Society" principle espoused by President Lyndon Johnson in the 1960s was a manifestation of a federal acceptance of responsibility for action to improve the lot of the poor and the disadvantaged in America's communities. On the other hand, the "New Federalism" of President Nixon, continued and accelerated by Presidents Carter and Reagan, reflected a desire to place greater responsibility on the individual and local community. The intent of regime policies by the latter presidents has been an overall decentralization of public control and responsibility, with a lessening of policy and program direction from the "federal pinnacle" of government. Consider the following statements of regime policy from the State of the Union addresses of Presidents Kennedy and Johnson.

> "A strong America depends on its cities--America's glory, and sometimes America's shame. To substitute sunlight for congestion and progress for decay, we have stepped up existing urban renewal and housing programs, and launched new ones--redoubled the attack on water pollution--speeded aid to airports, hospitals, highways, and our declining mass transit systems--and secured new weapons to combat organized crime, racketeering, and youth delinquency, assisted by the coordinated and hard-hitting efforts of our investigative services: the FBI, the Internal Revenue, the Bureau of Narcotics, and many others.

60

We shall need further anti-crime, mass transit, and transportation legislation--and new tools to fight air pollution."
                              -John F. Kennedy
                              January 11, 1962

"Let this session of Congress be known as the session which did more for civil rights than the last hundred sessions combined; as the session which enacted the most far-reaching tax cut of our time; as the session which declared all-out war on human poverty and unemployment in these United States; as the session which finally recognized the health needs of all our older citizens; as the session which reformed our tangled transportation and transit policies; as the session which achieved the most effective, efficient foreign aid program ever; and as the session which helped to build more homes, more schools, more libraries, and more hospitals than any single session of Congress in the history of our Republic."

                              . . .

"This budget, and this year's legislative program, are designed to help each and every American citizen fulfill his basic hopes--his hopes for a fair chance to make good; his hopes for fair play from the law; his hopes for a full-time job on full-time pay; his hopes for a decent home for his family in a decent community; his hopes for a good school for his children with good teachers; and his hopes for security when faced with sickness or unemployment or old age."
                              -Lyndon B. Johnson
                              January 8, 1964.

The statements above signaled the beginning of a decade of policies to promote individual and community well-being throughout America. Not fifteen years later, U.S. Presidents were signaling quite different directions for national leadership. Excerpts from State of the Union addresses of Presidents Carter and Reagan signal a policy of federal withdrawal from national responsibility for Americans and their communities.

". . . [there] is a limit to the role and the function of government. Government cannot solve our problems, it can't set our goals, it cannot define our vision. Government cannot eliminate poverty or provide a

61

bountiful economy or reduce inflation or save our cities or cure illiteracy or provide energy. And government cannot mandate goodness."
–Jimmy Carter
January 19, 1978

"[My] plan is based on our commonsense fundamentals: continued reduction of the growth in Federal spending; preserving the individual and business tax reductions that will stimulate saving and investment; removing unnecessary Federal regulations to spark productivity; and maintaining a healthy dollar. . . .

. . .

We must cut out more nonessential government spending and rout out more waste, and we will continue to reduce the number of employees in the Federal work force by 75,000.

The budget plan I submit to you on February 8th will realize major savings by dismantling the Departments of Energy and Education and by eliminating ineffective subsidies for business. We'll continue to redirect our resources to our two highest bedget priorities--a strong national defense to keep American free and at peace and a reliable safety net of social programs for those who have contributed and those who are in need.

Contrary to some of the wild charges you may have heard, this administration has not and will not turn its back on America's elderly or America's poor.

. . . We will protect them. But there's only one way to see to it that these programs really help those whom they were designed to help. And that is to bring their spiraling costs under control.

. . .

The time has come to control the uncontrollable. In August we made a start. I signed a bill to reduce the growth of these programs by $44 billion over the next 3 years while at the same time preserving essential services to the truly needy."
–Ronald Reagan
January 26, 1982

The concepts of "safety net" and "truly needy" signaled the intent of President Reagan's policy to reduce federal support for many programs which had been established for over two decades.

The regime policy of the Reagan administration is to shift toward reliance on the forces of a "market economy," and for private organizations and lower levels of government to accept responsibility for individual and community development. We see here two strains in the system of American values reflected in the regime policies of Presidents. The Kennedy and Johnson years were years of federal acceptance of social responsibility for our fellow Americans. The Carter and Reagan statements reflect the economic "survival of the fittest" values which place responsibility on individuals and localities for the well-being of themselves and their families.

Sectoral Public Policy--Or, Community Subsystem Policy

The first aspect of this third category of policy to be considered concerns the principles which guide public decision-makers in formulating laws and establishing programs to achieve social goals in specific areas. "Public policy" may involve both constraints **and** social purposes in relation to the behavior of citizens and their well-being. Morris has stated that, in this sense, public policy acts as a guide to the "aims of governing":

> [A] government must . . . decide to what extent it will regulate the acts of its citizens in order to pursue the goal of general well-being, to what extent it will direct its citizens to act in their private capacities to satisfy their own needs, or to what extent it will provide for citizens' needs directly through governmental agencies. (1979, p. 17)

Morris' statement can be dissected into three principal aspects of public policy. Each reflects an intent of government with respect to the "public" and its well-being. First, public policy may act to **regulate** behavior in an attempt to guard the individual and collective well-being of citizens or to advance goals of justice and equity. For example, current legislation restricting the release of pollutants into the atmosphere by automobiles and industrial plants, requirements for new drugs to be tested and approved before released for sale to the public, control of monopolistic practices in industry and business, and restrictions on the discretionary behavior of law enforcement officers with respect to suspects--all of these reflect the regulatory aspect of public policy.

Regulatory public policies, of course, are not restricted to the level of federal government. Corresponding public policies can also be found at the levels of state and local government. For example, a few states have anti-littering laws that require bottled beverages to be distributed in containers on which an initial deposit is made and can be later recovered when the container is returned to a dealer. Many municipalities have local ordinances requiring home owners to keep sidewalks free of snow in the wintertime, banning smoking in public buildings and some commercial establishments, and restricting the burning of trash or leaves in outdoor burners--all regulations designed as public safety measures. Both state and local governments have public health and sanitation laws covering publicly licensed food-serving establishments and other distributors of prepared foods. All of these are examples of public regulatory policies designed as measures for public safety and well-being.

The **second** aspect of public policy mentioned by Morris concerns a government's encouragement to its citizens to be self-reliant in satisfying many of their own needs. For example, gainful employment by individuals and the use of income from work to support self and family is, in effect, a widely accepted "public policy" stance in the United States. Governmental intervention in this area occurs only when the worker-job market relationship fails to function properly; for example, in cases of industrial accidents, prolonged layoff, death or disability of a household's primary wage earner, and the like. Individuals and heads of households are also presumed to be responsible for their own and their families' health needs through private insurance or through employer-provided health insurance plans. Again, governmental intervention occurs only when an individual's or household's income is insufficient to meet health care needs, as in cases of temporary or permanent disabilities, or the lack of income or private health insurance among many of the elderly. The principle of "self-reliance" is a firmly engrained value in the American social fabric, and, to the extent possible, it is "public policy" at each level of government to encourage and support citizens to meet their needs by private means. In recent years, for example, it has become public policy for federal, state, and local governments to encourage greater "private initiative" in the human services, principally through increased use of volunteers in social programs and improved private-public sector collaboration in dealing with many social issues, such as local industrial and labor-force development and provision of housing to low-income populations.

The **third** aspect of public policy identified by Morris provides for citizens' needs through public agencies and programs. It is at this point that we begin to encounter a number of apparent contradictions in public **social** policies in the United States. On the one hand, public social welfare policy is essentially "residual" in its orientation toward government's responsibilities, based on the presumption that dependence on public assistance in any form should be a "last resort option." At the same time, however, it has become increasingly evident that governmental intervention through social programs has become an important part of the public policy agenda since the time of the mid-1930s, and especially since the early 1960s. Such public policy goals as "eliminating poverty," "combatting illiteracy," and "assuring adequate health care to all citizens" exemplify recent national intentions that have transcended particular administrations and specific governmental jurisdictions. Admittedly, the commitment to these public policy goals and their implementation may vary among national administrations and other levels of government, but there is little doubt that they have emerged as ingredients of an agenda for governmental intervention in helping particular segments of the population and the general citizenry itself attain an adequate standard of living. Moreover, looked at analytically, they demonstrate an ever-increasing linkage between personal problems and public responses, which is the essence of social policy in the public arena.

Thus, public policy serves as a guide to the aims and priorities of governments--federal, state and local--with respect to the security and well-being of citizens within their jurisdictions. It provides signals to individual citizens and to organizations in both the public and the private sectors about what government and they should be trying to do, and where governmental intervention is likely to occur when behavior goes astray or when needs arise that simply can't be met through individual, private means.

Sectoral Social Policy

Public social policy can be separated into a number of **"sectoral"** policies (or "subsystem" policies), each dealing with a particular national, state, or local concern. For example, we can (and do) refer to health policy, welfare policy, housing policy, environmental policy, transportation policy, economic development policy, and employment and training policy, along with many others. In effect, each of these "policy sectors" comprises a relatively separate focus for social policy and program development in the United States, in that each typically affects only a segment of the society and is legislated and administered in a comparatively discrete fashion. At the federal level, for example, these various policy sectors are reflected in the several cabinet departments in the executive branch; for example, the Departments of Health and Human Services, Labor, Transportation, Housing and Urban Development, and Commerce.

Several commentators on social policy in the United States point to the existence of these sectors of social policy concern and the many social programs each encompasses as illustrating the lack of a national social policy of any meaningful sort. Moynihan, writing in 1970, noted that "the structure of American government, and the pragmatic tradition of American politics, too much defined public policy in the forms of **program,** and in consequence has inhibited the development of true **policy."** Moynihan was particularly critical of the "limitations of the **program** approach to issues which demand the disciplined formulations and elaborations of public **policy."** (Moynihan, 1972, p. 90) Macarov has also commented on the tendency in the United States to "partialize" social welfare concerns, focusing primarily on areas of specific concern, such as poverty, mental health, child care, and the like. (Macarov, 1978) The result of this "piecemeal" approach has been that all of these have become "value subsystems," with each providing a relatively distinct arena for policy development and a profusion of social programs for particularized problems in human development.

From the standpoint of local communities and their human services, sectoral policies and the programs they give rise to may be directed towards the needs of a specific segment of the local population (e.g., the elderly) or, in some instances, result in benefits to all local citizens (e.g., new public transportation facilities). Nonetheless, from the standpoint of social policy, both are expressions of **sectoral** policy. In either instance, the policy and program focus is on a specific group or aspect of the local community, thus dealing with only a "slice" of human development by linking personal and group needs to collective solutions in a narrowly limited way. For example, health care provided through public programs for low-income individuals and families may well affect the distribution of medical services among a community's population; that is one of its program and policy targets. However, it is not directly concerned with other issues of income maintenance or skills training and job placement of low-income individuals; these latter "belong" to other human service subsystems dealing with problems of income and employment and training development. This is not to say, however, that they are **not** interdependent, at least in ways unintended and perhaps not entirely visible to policy makers and program personnel in the various sectoral programs. For example, the quality of health and medical care may well affect the job readiness and later work performance of the low-income unemployed. But, as Moynihan notes, it is not rare to discover that the problems social policies should ostensibly cover are themselves systemically interrelated, though our piecemeal and fragmented responses through sectoral policies and categorical programs seldom take account of this interdependence. (Moynihan, 1972)

Below, several major sectoral social policy areas are described with respect to the principal underlying value and normative themes that give rise to human service programs in each area. It will be seen that, although each area is a source of policy intervention into the problems of individuals and groups, each deals with a relatively separate arena of community life--or, as noted earlier, just a "slice" of human development concern. One can also note the differences that exist among these several policy arenas, and the fact that the conflicts that exist about policy priorities are often manifest in laws, programs, and the behavior of various actors in different state and local community settings.

Health Care: Public policy generally endorses the idea that individuals and families should be responsible for obtaining necessary health care services in the marketplace. Certainly, there is no nationally supported health care system, although there are a number of programs for special groups, such as military veterans. There are also two federally supported insurance-type programs to aid the elderly (Medicare) and the poor (Medicaid) by paying for most, but not necessarily all, of their health and medical costs. Some states also have additional programs authorized by legislation, alongside their participation in the federal Medicaid program, to help lower-income elderly individuals and families deal with the costs of health care. For example, the State of Pennsylvania recently enacted legislation to use proceeds from the state lottery to assist elderly persons of limited means in paying for prescription medicines. (It might also be noted, though, that the State of Arizona elected not to participate with the federal government in the Medicaid program--an option to each of the states, since Medicaid is financed jointly by federal and state funds.)

Unless directly employed by a municipal, state or federal hospital, medical personnel offer services for a price in the marketplace. At the same time, private organizations such as professional medical societies have a strong influence on the availability and quality of care, subject to licensing requirements of state governments. However, communities frequently establish and support the hospitals wherein private professionals practice.

The dominant delivery system in the health care field involves medical treatment, although competing models exist including chiropractic, Christian Science, holistic health, acupuncture, and others. There are also other health care providers who are also closely associated with public social policy in this sector; for example, home health agencies, which are typically (but not always) private nonprofit organizations providing home care services supported both by direct fee-payers by third-party reimbursements from federal and state agencies, and by private insurance carriers.

Public Health: One of the principal policy themes in this subsystem area relates to the public's right to be protected from health hazards in the environment. Extensive responsibility for policy formulation and implementation is assigned to the public sector, involving all three levels of government--federal, state and local. Control of sewage and protection of water supplies, research into the nature of contagious diseases, and preventive health programs such as immunizations are regarded as **public** responsibilities. This is in addition to other public health services of a regulatory character, such as the testing and control of drugs and medicines offered by prescription or over-the-counter sales, food additives, and a host of other consumer products. In large measure, many of the preventive public health programs have become such everyday affairs in local community life that many citizens do not recognize the extent to which sectoral public policies in this area intervene in their lives and the life of their communities. For example, restaurants are inspected regularly by public health officers to see if they meet public standards of sanitation. Municipal code enforcement officials examine private dwellings and commercial buildings for compliance with public fire and safety codes.

Human-produced pollutants and their release into the environment are, of course, concerns of more recent vintage. Such concerns relate to air quality, as well as to stewardship of lands and waterways. These are problem areas in which a great amount of conflict has emerged with respect to competing values in American society: on the one hand, advocates of clean air and water, and the restoration of ravaged terrains caused by surface mining and clean-cut logging; and, on the other, advocates of the rights of industry to exploit available natural resources and to utilize the most efficient production technologies, claiming both as essential to the general economic welfare of American society. In this particular domain of public health policy, many issues continue to be hotly debated, and thus far the outcomes have been a series of compromises between the two sets of advocates.

Mental Health Care: Publicly supported mental health services are generally provided through state or local mental hospitals, or through local community mental health centers and their contracted service providers. Private mental health care is also available through individual practitioners and privately operated mental hospitals and clinics. The notion of "mental health" encompasses a broad array of individual problems with emotional well-being. The developmentally disabled are also frequently included in the mental health "target population."

The movement towards **community** mental health centers and facilities is a relatively recent development in the United States, only getting underway with any force with the passage of the Community Mental Health Centers Act in 1963. Since the 1963 act's passage, there have been competing ideas in the field, some stressing community-based care for larger portions of the general public in accordance with a "right to treatment" ideology, and others believing that community mental health services are much overrated as needed community services. Additionally, there have been the strains within the mental health profession arising from the drive to "deinstitutionalize" the mentally ill and find acceptable care for them within local communities, not institutions. (Mental hospitals have come under increasing criticism as "warehouses" for the mentally ill, providing them little in the way of rehabilitative treatment and care.)

If one looks closely at the history of social values in the United States and their effects on the development of public social policies, public responsibility for the mentally ill and others whose mental incompetence has prevented them from achieving independent living styles has been fairly strong, particularly over the last century. Currently, however, the debate has shifted, as ideas regarding what constitutes mental "illness" have changed. For example, is the stress experienced by a long-term unemployed worker an issue of public mental health concern? How questions such as this are answered is a strong determinant of the extent to which publicly supported mental health services are extended to ever-increasing numbers of citizens, regardless of background or income level.

Criminal Justice: Public security and police services have long been recognized as public responsibilities. However, public policy in the area of criminal justice is often beset by two competing sets of principles. One emphasizes the public's right to protection from the illegal acts of others: apprehension, trial, conviction and punishment of criminal offenders are stressed. In short, for the security and general well-being of the law-abiding public, offenders should be isolated through incarceration.

The other set of principles emphasizes the rights of citizens and seeks to protect them from unreasonable acts by governmental agents responsible for the **administration** of justice (courts, police, probation and parole, corrections). The assurance of "due process" rights, guaranteed by the Constitution, and the avoidance of abuse and harassment by public officials in the justice system make up the essential platform of this second set of principles.

Conflict over these two dominant sets of policy principles are manifest daily on the streets of local communities, in precinct houses, in the courts, and in legislatures. This conflict is exacerbated by the current controversy over whether criminals should be punished or provided rehabilitative treatment while incarcerated. There is probably no other public social policy sector, unless it should be that of juvenile justice, in which value conflicts swing to and fro to such an extent, influencing public policy first in one direction and then another.

Juvenile Justice: Young people below the age of majority are not considered to be fully responsible for their actions. Thus, public policy in the United States has assigned primary responsibility for their socialization and control to families and community institutions, such as the schools. In recent years, public policy in juvenile justice has been based on the principle that the long-range, best interests of children and youth are served by providing for their habilitation and/or rehabilitation. The policy focus is not on punishment for a law-violating act, but rather on what might be needed to help the youngster grow into a mature, responsible adult.

As a result of this predominant policy principle, rehabilitative services in a "family court" setting prevail in the area of juvenile justice. Due process rights and punishment are most often considered to interfere with effective treatment and are thus deemphasized--although since the **In Re Gault** court decision in 1967, juvenile courts have been much more limited in overlooking or bypassing the due process rights of juveniles appearing before the court. Within the juvenile justice system, however, conflict continues to occur over the issues of "punishment and penitence" vs. rehabilitation and movement toward adult maturity and responsibility.

Children and Youth: Young people are valued members of any local community, as they are of the larger society. Dominant social values prescribe that they should be cared for, nurtured and educated, so that they can grow to mature, responsible adulthood. Primary responsibility for this correct nurturance rests with parents and relatives. However, the **parens patriae** doctrine (the state as higher parent) prescribes community (public) intervention if parents or relatives fail to shoulder their responsibilities properly by neglecting or abusing their children.

Both the abused or neglected child, and the developmentally disabled child, are seen through the eye of public policy as deserving of special attention by the society and community. Competing policy perspectives in this area would, on the one hand, expand the **parens patriae** doctrine to include public intervention for mental as well as physical abuse, and for cultural and educational deficiencies. Moreover, there is a continuing, almost raging, public debate over the provision of planned parenthood services and birth control counseling for teenagers. And, of course, many of the due process concerns within the juvenile justice system for alleged delinquents also carry over into the dependent-child area.

Income Maintenance: As noted earlier, it is a strongly held value in American society that individuals should be responsible for their own physical and material well-being through productive, gainful employment and purchase of goods and services in the marketplace. This, of course, is a policy principle that is not seen as applying in the case of "vulnerable" populations, such as the elderly, the deserted wife and children, and the physically and mentally disabled. Since the time of the passage of the Elizabethan Poor Law in 1601, a distinction has been made between the "deserving" and "nondeserving" poor in the formulation of public policies regarding the awarding of public assistance in the form of income maintenance. The "poor law" philosophy still largely sets the terms of public debate in the United States about income maintenance programs, even though there is increasing evidence that more and more of the American population is tending toward an attitude that "deservingness" is something more than a temporary condition; for example, that the displaced worker in the steel industry who cannot find employment after months of job seeking is just as "deserving" of public assistance in income maintenance as the non-working widow with dependent-age children.

Within the United States, since the time of the 1930s we have had two types of income maintenance programs--called by Steiner "crude" and "subtle" relief. (Steiner, 1971) "Crude" relief refers to the typical public assistance program, presumably reserved for the "deserving poor" as depicted in the Elizabethan Poor Law statutes. "Subtle" relief is something else. It primarily refers to income maintenance programs publicly advanced as "entitlement" programs, such as Social Security retirement income and unemployment compensation. Both of these latter programs have been touted as "social insurance" programs, though neither is. Social Security retirement benefits are the products of an "income transfer" program; in effect, taking from the pocket of those currently employed (and their employers) and placing the transferred dollars into the pocket of the eligible retiree. Granted, during his or her working lifetime, the beneficiary paid into the Social Security fund, as did employers, but in no sense can Social Security (formally, Old Age, Survivors and Disability Insurance) be regarded as a "true" social insurance program. Similarly, unemployment compensation is funded by contributions of an individual's employer on a regular (payday) basis. What an unemployed individual receives from the unemployment compensation fund depends on his/her work record over a specified period of time; in effect, the more consistent and stable the work record, the higher the level of unemployment benefits.

The area of income maintenance policies is probably the most hotly debated of the sectoral policy areas. On the one hand, there are those who assert the right to a decent standard of living and guaranteed annual income for all Americans, regardless of physical, mental, or age status. On the other hand, there are those who would sharply restrict income maintenance support programs, both in terms of the eligible populations for public assistance and in the amount and duration of the aid given.

Housing: Home ownership, particularly the single-family dwelling, has long been an American ideal. Moreover, dominant social values promote the responsibility of individuals (and their families) to secure their own shelter in the marketplace of the private economy. At the same time, several national administrations, beginning with President Eisenhower in the 1950s, have espoused the general policy goal of "decent housing for all Americans." This policy goal has been pursued primarily through three means: government-supported loans to military veterans; income-tax breaks to any American with a qualifying mortgage interest deduction; and subsidized public rental units for the poor and elderly. (For example,

Section 8 of the federal Housing Act of 1974 authorized the Department of Housing and Urban Development to enter into rental contracts with housing owners to provide "guaranteed rent" services to low-income families. In effect, Section 8 provides for the HUD-based program to make up the difference between a "fair market rent" and approximately 20% of the low-income occupant's monthly household income.)

Economic and Community Development: Fundamental American values have always favored support of private parties to develop the nation. Land grants to nobles by European aristocracies provided incentives to encourage colonists to settle in the New World. Homesteading and squatters' rights extended the idea to millions of individuals. Grants of land to railroads and mining interests also had the objective of fostering the development of the nation. Vast areas of federal land in the West are still leased to ranchers to use as their own; and mineral and oil exploration is encouraged by governmental leasing policies.

American values tend to emphasize the right to use one's land as one wishes. However, zoning and land-use policies allow communities to place some restrictions on owners in the broader public interest. More recently there has emerged a concern for the quality of life in our cities and towns. There is a consequent shift toward values which stress the quality of social, cultural and economic life as well as the physical characteristics of urban and community life. Community goal-setting and planning provide broad-based perspectives on how land and properties may be used, and incentives for specific types of development.

Current issues in this arena address, first, the use of the public environment for private purposes: oil and mineral exploitation and use of public lands for private profits raise questions of equity, fairness, and conservation for future generations. Secondly, the extent to which the public should be involved in controlling and improving the quality of urban life is a volatile issue. The proper locus of responsibility, and the extent to which private developers should be subject to public restrictions are issues which remain unsettled. Third, many state and local governments have policies designed to stabilize and improve local economies through industrial development. These policies typically contain both financial incentives and regulatory features intended to make the locality an attractive site for business operations. Local economic development efforts typically have three/aims: the retention of existing business and industries; encouragement of local entrepeneurs, who may extend existing product lines or develop entirely new local establishments; and, the attraction of new business and industrial firms to the local area. The issue of limiting or encouraging growth is one which confronts every American community today.

Public Policy and Change

Sectoral public policy principles provide definite parameters for decisionmaking and action. They both establish guidelines for the development of more specific goals and laws, and they offer targets for change. Cooperation is frequently nurtured among groups that agree on fundamental values. Conflict arises when groups differ on subsystem principles, and when policies based on these principles are advocated.

Sectoral value subsystem policies permeate all levels and jurisdictions in America. These policy areas provide broad guides for decisionmaking and action at federal, state and local levels, and they are manifest in the public, voluntary and private sectors of action. The specific manifestations in communities, however, vary both over time and in different jurisdictions. The next category of our typology addresses differences in policies as enacted into law and regulations by specific jurisdictions.

Jurisdictional Policy

"Jurisdictional policy and law" refers specifically to policies as espoused, intended, or enacted into laws by particular organizational jurisdictions. "Jurisdiction" connotes the area over which a particular individual actor or organization has authority. Generally, jurisdiction refers to a territory within a governing or ruling body, such as a state, city, county or township government; or a private corporate domain, which may be subdivided into regions, districts or units. Jurisdictional coverage may be general, as over all aspects of policy in a territory or domain, or it may be specifically restricted to a particular topic, such as child welfare, juvenile justice, health or housing in the public sector, or employment, personnel, wages, or product presentation in the private sector. Although a later chapter in this book will examine the various levels and sectors of jurisdictions as these exist in the United States, it is important at this point to recognize the distinction between two dimensions of jurisdiction. On the one hand, there is the dimension of **public-sector** involvement, which includes federal, state, and local governments. On the other, there is the dimension of **private-sector** involvement, which encompasses all nongovernmental entities, those within the voluntary nonprofit sector, and others within the sector of private business and industrial corporations. Throughout this discussion it is important to remember that **jurisdictional policy** is also subject to principles of the sectoral value subsystem arenas of policy discussed earlier.

There is considerable variation among states and localities as to how the jurisdictional policies and the programs they give rise to are defined. For example, in the area of federally assisted programs for income maintenance, which are combined federal-state funded programs, there are notable differences among the states as to the average monthly benefits paid to public assistance recipients. Note in Figure 2.1 that in 1981, average monthly payments per recipient in the Aid to Families with Dependent Children (AFDC) ranged from highs of $634 in Alaska and $601 in California for a family of four, to $148 in Alabama and $120 in Mississippi among the fifty states. (Social Security Bulletin, 1982, p. 263). The variations in jurisdictional policy, laws and programs are so vast that we shall not attempt to describe them at this point. Later chapters will allow the reader to examine some of the jurisdictional differences which American citizens confront.

Administrative Policy

The general policies and laws of specific jurisdictions are typically referred to administative units within the jurisdictional organization for translation and implementation. It is often necessary for the latter organizations to promulgate more specific guides to

Figure 2.1

Characteristics of State Plans for Aid to Families with Dependent Children

AMOUNTS FOR ALL BASIC NEEDS, AS DEFINED BY STATE NEED STANDARDS, AND AMOUNTS OF PAYMENT TO FAMILIES WITH NO COUNTABLE INCOME, AFTER APPLICATION OF ANY STATE PAYMENT LIMITATIONS, AS OF OCTOBER 1, 1981

(Rounded to the next highest dollar)

State	Family of Two Persons (One Needy Adult and One Child)		Family of Four Persons (One Needy Adult and Three Children)	
	State Need Standard for All Basic Needs	Amount of Assistance Payment to a Family With No Income	State Need Standard for All Basic Needs	Amount of Assistance Payment to a Family With No Income
Alabama	$288.00	$ 89.00	$480.00	$148.00
Alaska	508.00	508.00	634.00	634.00
Arizona	180.00	156.00	282.00	244.00
Arkansas	193.00	100.00	273.00	142.00
California	408.00	408.00	601.00	601.00
Colorado[1]	247.00	247.00	379.00	379.00
Connecticut	347.00	347.00	501.00	501.00
Delaware	197.00	197.00	312.00	312.00
D.C.	311.00	225.00	481.00	349.00
Florida	150.00	150.00	230.00	230.00
Georgia	306.00	153.00	432.00	216.00
Guam	195.00	195.00	300.00	300.00
Hawaii	390.00	390.00	546.00	546.00
Idaho	446.00	245.00	627.00	345.00
Illinois	326.00	235.00	581.00	349.00
Indiana	247.00	195.00	363.00	315.00
Iowa	292.00	292.00	419.00	419.00
Kansas	272.00	272.00	374.00	374.00
Kentucky	162.00	162.00	235.00	235.00
Louisiana	331.00	137.00	565.00	234.00
Maine	307.00	223.00	522.00	378.00
Maryland	211.00	211.00	326.00	326.00
Massachusetts	314.00	314.00	445.00	445.00
Michigan[2]	357.00	357.00	508.00	508.00
Minnesota	368.00	368.00	520.00	520.00

[1] Effective 12/1/81, the amounts for basic needs and amount of payment become $247 for two; $379 for four.
[2] Effective 12/1/81, the amount of payment becomes $327 for two; $465 for four.

State	Family of Two Persons (One Needy Adult and One Child)		Family of Four Persons (One Needy Adult and Three Children)	
	State Need Standard for All Basic Needs	Amount of Assistance Payment to a Family With No Income	State Need Standard for All Basic Needs	Amount of Assistance Payment to a Family With No Income
Mississippi	$188.00	$ 60.00	$252.00	$120.00
Missouri	250.00	199.00	365.00	290.00
Montana	311.00	233.00	473.00	355.00
Nebraska	280.00	280.00	420.00	420.00
Nevada	229.00	211.00	341.00	341.00
New Hampshire	292.00	292.00	392.00	392.00
New Jersey	273.00	273.00	414.00	414.00
New Mexico	189.00	189.00	281.00	281.00
New York	356.00	356.00	515.00	515.00
North Carolina	334.00	167.00	420.00	210.00
North Dakota[1]	270.00	408.00	270.00	408.00
Ohio	346.00	215.00	515.00	319.00
Oklahoma	218.00	218.00	349.00	349.00
Oregon	286.00	286.00	409.00	409.00
Pennsylvania	273.00	273.00	395.00	395.00
Puerto Rico	132.00	66.00	228.00	114.00
Rhode Island	298.00	298.00	420.00	420.00
South Carolina	144.00	102.00	229.00	163.00
South Dakota	280.00	280.00	361.00	361.00
Tennessee	142.00	97.00	217.00	148.00
Texas	122.00	85.00	201.00	141.00
Utah	407.00	279.00	640.00	438.00
Vermont	626.00	432.00	842.00	581.00
Virgin Islands	154.00	154.00	263.00	263.00
Virginia	201.00	181.00	314.00	283.00
Washington	361.00	361.00	515.00	515.00
West Virginia	219.00	164.00	332.00	249.00
Wisconsin	472.00	401.00	662.00	563.00
Wyoming[2]	280.00	280.00	340.00	340.00

[1] Effective 11/1/81, the amounts for basic needs and amount of payment become $289 for two and $437 for four.
[2] Effective 11/1/81, the amounts for basic needs and amount of payment become $320 for two and $390 for four.

action, in order to direct and control the uniformity and accountability of subsequent service delivery operations. Thus, administrative guidelines elaborate policies and laws into more detailed and specific directions and procedures for service delivery.

Within the area of public assistance programs, for example, federal policy mandates that participating states establish a "standard level" for its federally assisted cash assistance programs. In the State of Pennsylvania, the law requires that the "minimum level of health and decency" be provided to "all the needy and distressed." However, the "standard" for determining what aid will actually be provided within Pennsylvania was developed by the State Department of Public Welfare, not the legislature. Furthermore, administrative regulations specify the criteria which a person must meet in order to qualify for public aid. While these rules are subject to legislative "oversight," in reality considerable discretionary authority is delegated to the administering units--in this case, the Pennsylvania Department of Public Welfare. (In fact, some observers have noted the emergence of "new law" in situations where elaborate regulations and administrative guidelines have led to considerably expanded, restricted or distorted practice when compared to what was originally intended by the higher levels of legislative or executive authorization.)

Such administrative policies and regulations provide the formal (typically written and published) basis on which local community and human service agencies operate. Extensive "manuals" of regulations make explicit the requirements of programs and the constraints under which human service professionals work. The criteria of need, level of benefits, procedures for application and qualification, service delivery and evaluation are frequently lengthy and detailed. Supervision and accountability by higher levels of authority are based on comparison of actual performance to the standards established in administrative regulations and procedures.

Delivery- Or Street-Level Policy And Procedure

Perhaps the most specific level of policy in the areas of human development and human services occurs at the point of service delivery. "Policy" at this point is seldom formal or written, though it does reflect the difference between street-level units (or front-line workers) in the application of administrative policies and regulations.

Every set of laws or regulations necessarily leaves a degree of discretion to those who must implement them. Moreover, the ability to supervise and control subordinates is most often far from total. Individual workers in the human services agency have, or can take, different degrees of freedom in delivering services. Moreover, such workers are frequently subject to pressures from within as well as outside the organization to deviate from written, formal policy.

Discretionary authority for street-level workers may be necessary and even intentional within public policy. Police officers, for example, have considerable discretion in deciding where to patrol, whom to apprehend, and whom to actually arrest. Social workers necessarily must have considerable discretion in deciding whether physical punishment of a child is "abuse." Health professionals must make decisions about the level and nature of care and treatment. Discretionary authority is sometimes usurped by workers. Red tape, inflexibility, and excessive formalization of service delivery frequently lead to the effective denial of services to people who are in need and who, by objective criteria, qualify for services. While higher levels of authority are responsible for assuring that policies and laws are implemented, bureaucratic pressures frequently lead to a considerably less-than-perfect operation. Consider the following observation by Lipsky:

> Street-level bureaucrats are widely thought to lack sufficient organizational resources to accomplish their jobs. Classrooms are overcrowded. Large welfare caseloads prevent investigators from providing all but the cursory service. The lower courts are so overburdened that judges may spend their days adjourning but never trying cases. Police forces are perpetually understaffed, particularly as perceptions of crime and demands for civic order increase.
>
> Insufficiency of organizational resources increases the pressures on street-level bureaucrats to make quick decisions about clients and process cases with

inadequate information and too little time to dispose of problems on their merits. . . . The stakes are often high-- both to citizen and to bureaucrat. (Lipsky, 1972, pp. 171, 173)

Usurpation of authority in the opposite direction may occur as well. The concept of "client advocacy" is frequently used to justify evading or ignoring administrative policies and rules. This phenomenon occurs when workers decide that a "higher principle," such as the "Brother's Keeper" ethic or humanistic values, justifies the avoidance or conscious non-application of certain policies. Thus human service workers who know that the current welfare grant is well below the amount necessary for a particular family, may ignore small amounts of property or income which would reduce a public assistance grant. These "bandits in the bureaucracy" are, in effect, taking the law into their own hands to provide a different level of service than prescribed by policy. One worker in a Mobilization for youth program in New York put it this way:

When I think that Mrs. Cortez hasn't gotten any money for her rat allowance I sometimes want to throw up my hands and say: What difference does it make? Why should people in this day and age have rat allowances. . . . But when I realize that it isn't just the rat allowance . . . that it's a total system of oppressiveness and disrespect for people, why then I've got to get her that rat allowance. I've got to help her get as many things as possible. (Cloward and Elman, 1974, p. 208)

This most specific, "grassroots," level of policy determines the quality and character of service delivery at the point of action. Implementation of the most grandiose policies by community systems is dependent in the final analysis on the actions of street-level workers. The personal values and ethics of workers, and the professional standards they practice, will determine the outcome of higher levels of policy and authority. This personal level of the service delivery worker is analogous at the lowest level of the policy system to "regime policy" at the higher levels. As **regime policy** reflects the personal policy of a leader or set of leaders, so **street-**

level policy reflects the personal policy of a worker or group of workers.

Policies And Systems

The typology of policies we have presented provides an initial framework for understanding the character and operation of human services programs in the United States, especially as they are implemented in local community environments. The typology moves from the very general to the very specific. More specific types of policy provide guidance for subsystems concerned with particular areas of individual and collective life: health, housing, welfare and justice, for example. Sectoral policies devolve into jurisdictional policies and laws, administrative regulations and procedures, and are ultimately implemented by street-level workers. Flexibility and discretion exist at all levels, leading to differences in policy application. **Policies reflect the principles and rules which both facilitate and constrain the operation of community and human services systems.** The next chapter introduces the concept of "systems," and applies it to policymaking and action in the human services area.

Chapter II

REFERENCES

Anderson, James. **Public Policy-Making.** New York: Praeger, 1975.

Bannister, Robert C. **American Values in Transition.** New York: Harcourt, Brace, Jovanovitch, 1972.

Barnum, Phineas T. "The Art of Money Getting," in **Struggles and Triumphs.** 1879.

Burke, Edmund. **Reflections on the Revolution in France.** Chicago, III.: Henry Regnery Company, 1955.

Cloward, Richard R., and Richard E. Elman, "Advocacy in the Ghetto," in Fred M. Cox et al., eds. **Strategies of Community Organization.** Itasca, III.: F. E. Peacock Publishers, 1974.

Dictionary of Social Science, ed. John T. Zadrozny. Washington, D.C.: Public Affairs Press, 1959.

Dorsen, Norman, ed. **The Rights of Americans: What They Are--What They Should Be.** New York:: Pantheon Books, 1971.

Easton, David. **The Political System.** 2nd ed. New York: Alfred A. Knopf, 1971.

Edwards, George C. III, and Ira Sharkansky. **The Policy Predicament.** San Francisco: W. H. Freeman and Co., 1978.

Emerson, Thomas I., and David Haber. **Political and Civil Rights in the United States.** Buffalo, N.Y.: Dennis and Co., 1952.

Gabriel, Ralph H. **The Course of American Democratic Thought.** 2nd ed. New York: The Ronald Press Co., 1956.

Gil, David G. **Unravelling Social Policy.** 2nd ed. Cambridge, Mass.: Schenkman Publishing Company, Inc., 1981.

Goodman, Paul. **Growing Up Absurd.** N.Y.: Random House 1960.

Heclo, H. Hugh. "Policy Analysis." **British Journal of Political Science,** 2, January 1972.

Huttman, Elizabeth D. **Introduction to Social Policy.** New York: McGraw Hill Publishing Co., Inc., 1981.

Jenkins, W. I. **Policy Analysis.** New York: St. Martin's Press, 1978.

Katkin, Daniel, John Kramer and Drew Hyman. "Three Models of Juvenile Justice." **Criminal Law Bulletin,** 12, March-April 1976, 165-188.

Kennan, George F. "Rebels Without a Program," in **Democracy and the Student Left.** Boston, Ma.: Little, Brown and Co., 1968.

Lipsky, Michael. "Street-Level Bureaucracy and the Analysis of Urban Reform," in **Blacks and Bureaucracy,** ed. Virginia Ermer and John Strange. New York: Thomas Y. Crowell, Inc., 1972.

Lipsky, Michael. **Street-Level Bureaucracy: Dilemmas of the Individual in Public Services.** New York: Russell Sage Foundation, 1980.

Macarov, David. **Work and Welfare: The Unholy Alliance.** Beverly Hills, Calif.: Sage Publications, Inc., 1980.

Macarov, David. **The Design of Social Welfare.** New York: Holt, Rinehart, and Winston, 1978.

Marine, Gene. "America the Raped." **Ramparts.** Vol. 5, April-May, 1967.

Matthew, The Gospel According to. **The Holy Bible.** Revised Standard Version, N.Y.: Thomas Nelson & Sons, 1946, Chapter 25, Vs. 31-39.

Moynihan, Daniel P. "Policy vs. Program in the '70's." **The Public Interest,** 20, Summer, 1970, 90-100.

Morris, Robert. **Social Policy of the American Welfare State.** New York: Harper and Row, 1979.

Policy Studies Organization. **Policy Studies Journal.** Vol. 1, Autumn 1972.

President's Commission on Civil Rights. Washington, D.C.: U. S. Government Printing Office, 1947.

Steiner, Gilbert Y. **The State of Welfare.** Washington, D.C.: The Brookings Institution, 1971.

Sumner, Charles. "The Law of Human Progress." **Complete Works, Vol. II.** Boston, Ma.: Lee and Shepard 1900, p. 241-290.

Thoreau, Henry David. "Life Without Principle." **The Writings of Henry David Thoreau.** N.Y.: Powgen Press, 1936.

Washington, Booker Taliaferro. **Sowing and Reaping.** Freeport, N.Y.: Books for Libraries Press, 1971, reprint of the 1900 edition.

Weber, Max. **The Methodology of the Social Sciences,** tr. Edward A. Shils and Henry A. Finch. New York: The Free Press, 1949.

Webster's New World Dictionary, College Edition. Springfield, Mass.: G. & C. Merriam Company, 1973.

Zastrow, Charles. **Introduction to Social Welfare Institutions.** Homewood, Ill.: The Dorsey Press, 1978.

Chapter III

ON SYSTEMS IN GENERAL

"Find out the cause of this effect, or rather say, the cause of this defect, for this effect defective comes by cause."

—Hamlet, Act II, Sc. 2

Getting Into Systems Thinking

Policies occur in systems. Policies result from the plans and actions of systems. And policies affect the management and operation of systems. While we are concerned most specifically about the highly complex structures and interactions in American communities which we call "human service systems," it is important first to gain a fundamental understanding of systems in general. In this chapter we will consider some general principles of systems thinking. Definitions of fundamental concepts will provide tools for comparative understanding of many types of systems. Finally, we will present models of several community and human service systems to provide a transition to the application of systems thinking to human services. The result will be the initiation of a systematic way of looking at empirical phenomena, and a framework for understanding the highly interdependent and complex nature of human service systems.

Systems Thinking And You

Systems thinking is not difficult. You do it all the time. Consider yourself walking into your favorite "96-Flavors" ice cream store. They have a new product--frozen yogurt. "What's that?" you ask. "Frozen yogurt," the attendant says. "It's like ice cream, but it's supposed to have less calories and more nutrition."

"SYSTEMS THINKING BEGINS WITH A DESIRE TO KNOW ABOUT SOMETHING: WHAT IT IS FOR, AND HOW IT IS MADE UP."

"What's in it?" you ask. "How do they make it?" "You know," says the attendant, "they mix up a lot of things like fruit, sugar, yogurt, and stuff." "Like making ice cream, except you use yogurt instead of milk and cream." "Yogurt is a cultured milk product which provides more protein and less cholesterol." "Here, have a taste, then you can decide if you want this or our regular product."

"SYSTEMS THINKING INVOLVES A CONCERN FOR THE PARTS --AND THE WHOLE--AND HOW THEY WORK TOGETHER."

The above interaction has all the ingredients of systems thinking. There was a concern for understanding the **units,** the **process** of mixing or interaction, the purpose or **goal,** the nature of the overall product or **system,** and consideration of **options.** These are keys to systems thinking. As we said above, you do it all the time--implicitly. Now we want to have you learn to consciously use systems thinking as a way of understanding and analyzing events around you.

Begin focusing on questions about systems: What is interacting? On whom or what? By whom? In what ways? With what results? We begin with basic principles and everyday illustrations, and move toward more complex applications. You are asked to become aware of your intuitive understanding of systems in order to explicitly seek a better understanding of social policies, and to make decisions about how to improve community systems and human services.

>>NOTE: From time to time we shall reach out and "tap you on the shoulder" like this--to ask you to pause and think about an issue and to

consider your personal experiences.

Right now, for example, consider your goals for reading this book. What do you want to get out of it? How will you approach learning? How will it relate to what you already know? To your future career?<<

Systems Thinking As A Frame Of Reference

Social reality is an incredibly complicated web of interactions, each strand of which affects and is affected by many others. The direction of science in the 19th and 20th centuries has been toward specialization, that is, towards increasingly detailed examination of single strands, or even parts of single strands. Experts devote lifetimes to isolating and studying small aspects of a highly dynamic and interrelated reality. Each group of scientists, each discipline, and each profession has developed its theories and concepts to explain the nature and operation of selected aspects of human existence. These specializations have provided a greater reservoir of knowledge than has ever before been available to human beings, but much of the accumulated knowledge of the centuries is carried by different people; or, it is neatly stacked on shelves in thousands of libraries, isolated between the covers of millions of separate books.

Many of these sources have bits of information which are essential if we are to gain a more systematic understanding of human services policy and community systems. But the separate fields, or disciplines, have generally not attempted to interrelate the bits and pieces of knowledge into a broader, more understandable whole. This book asks you to begin to develop a picture of the broader complexity of social events. Systems thinking is a new way of looking at the world--a frame of reference which directs one's attention not just to the parts of reality, but also to the interactions of the parts in order to make it possible at some point to connect the parts. Systems thinking stresses the emergence of whole pictures.

Key Principles Of Systems Thinking

As you begin thinking about putting pieces together to make a larger whole, you address the key principle in systems thinking:

**"EVERY PORTION OF KNOWN EXISTENCE
CAN BE CONCEIVED OF AS SYSTEM:
AS SYSTEM WITHIN SYSTEM AND SYSTEM BEYOND SYSTEM."**

Think for a moment about putting together a jigsaw puzzle. Begin with many separate, individual pieces. You examine each piece carefully, but then you go on to ask questions about the relationship of each piece to all the others. The design and coloration of one piece is not merely interesting in its own right; it is significant because it suggests that there is a relationship with other pieces. The character of **and** your knowledge of others suggest where they fit together, or do not fit with other pieces. The information you get from each part of the puzzle constitutes a clue about the nature of other parts.

Systems thinking is a way of approaching knowledge as pieces of reality and asking about each one, "How does this fit with other things I know?" "What does this suggest about the larger picture?" "What clues does it give me about the nature of the whole web of relationships?"

The utility of systems thinking is that it asks you to develop pictures that are interdisciplinary and comprehensive. The overall picture of a jigsaw puzzle emerges only when the pieces are put together in a special way. Similarly, looking at the components of complex social and human service systems one at a time is hardly the best way to develop comprehensive understanding.

Conversely, though, it is very difficult to juggle more than a few sets of observations and concepts at the same time. As human beings we simply do not have the capacity to study dozens of different issues simultaneously. Thus, our study of complex interactions must be conducted in such a way as to consider the individual parts, but also to consider how they interrelate into a broader whole.

A corollary of the above principle is that **the universe as a system is ultimately made up of the interaction of its parts, and that each of the parts is affected in some way by others.** You are a system. You are part of other systems. You are also made up of many systems. In the universe, we can discern many types, sizes, levels, and components of systems. Consider atoms. Atoms are extremely small, sub-microscopic systems comprised of protons, neutrons, and other particles which interact according to discernible laws or rules. Somewhat larger molecules are comprised of interacting atoms. Molecules may combine to form cells . . . cells to form organs . . . and organs to form animals . . . some of which are human beings . . . which leads us to another principle of systems thinking:

"A SYSTEM IS ALWAYS EMBEDDED IN A LARGER SYSTEM"

You, for example, are part of a family system, an educational system, a community system, a social system, and economic, cultural, justice, political, and other systems. As with the jigsaw puzzle, each part can be viewed separately or in relation to the overall picture. A corollary principle of systems thinking is:

"A SYSTEM IS MADE UP OF SMALLER SYSTEMS."

As an individual you are made up of circulatory, respiratory, muscular, lymphatic, nervous, psychological, spiritual, motivational, and mental systems. You may not have thought about yourself in exactly this way before, but you are also made up of the economic, social, family, political and other systems of which you are a part. You would not be you without them. You would be a different person, a different system, and your future would be radically different if your environmental systems were different--which brings us to yet another principle of systems thinking:

"A SYSTEM IS MADE UP FROM ITS ENVIRONMENT."

Consider an unborn infant. It is part of its mother in whose womb it lives. It is also made up of nutrients from the mother's biological systems. From the moment of conception, a developing system exists which grows by interchange of nutrients and waste with the environment--the womb. This growing biological system is totally "made up" (created) from its environment. Furthermore, at birth (perhaps before) other people become involved and the psychological and reactive subsystems begin to develop by interchange of perceptions and actions. After birth, continued growth is dependent on interchanges with the environment--the parents, family, house, furniture, dog, peers, church, etc. Neither the emerging being nor the environment is the same from the point of the initial joining together of the sperm and ovum in the womb; and that joining together is an interaction between environmental systems.

>>Go back and reconsider the last four principles in the light of your own existence, and the relationship to others and to your environment. What might be the case if just one major variable were different?<<

Defining Systems

The preceding principles are important for understanding the nature of systems and interactional causation. A "system" is most fundamentally a series of smaller entities, or units, in more or less regular interaction. The action of the system is "caused" by the interaction of the units with each other and with environmental systems. We will have more to say later about this theory of causation, but first we are ready for a few definitions of systems.

[A system is] (1) a set of elements, (2) the relationship between and among the elements, and (3) the notion of movement in unison in obedience to some form of control . . . some ongoing process of a set of elements each of which are functionally and operationally united in the achievement of an objective.

−S. L. Optner

A system is a set of objects together with relationships between the objects and between their attributes.

−Hall and Fagen

A system is a set or arrangement of things so related or connected as to form a unity or organic whole: as, a solar system . . . the world . . . the body considered as a functioning organism.

−Webster's New World Dictionary

A SET OF UNITS WITH RELATIONSHIPS AMONG THEM.

−Ludwig von Bertalanffy

Two fundamental characteristics of any system are (1) that it has differentiated parts and (2) that its parts are interdependent.

−James D. Thompson

A system is, roughly speaking, a bundle of relationships.

-Anatol Rapoport

A SYSTEM IS A COLLECTION OF INTERACTING SYSTEMS.

-John Beckett

From these definitions, it is clear that a system consists of some things variously called **objects, units, actors, components, variables, or elements.** And these units must **interact . . . have relationships between them** . . . and be interconnected or interdependent . . . for a system to exist. Moreover, when a system operates, the units in interaction do something which is variously called **purpose, goal, function, effect, or output.** In order to produce the action or output, there are some **rules** or **processes** which govern the interactions. These comments lead us to a further, and very basic, principle of systems.

"A SYSTEM IS MORE THAN THE SUM OF ITS PARTS."

Consider a watch. Dismantled, it is a pile of gears, screws, pins, springs--a pile of metal objects and jewels. The hands do not turn. There is neither "tick" nor "tock." Silence. Stillness. A watch is **more than** its parts--it is those parts involved in a regular and ongoing set of relationships. Think about other systems--yourself, a car, a factory, a hospital. It is not just the parts that make them what they are--active, productive systems--but also the interactions among the parts. The interactions constitute the system **"process,"** an important concept for you to remember.

As process is important in determining the fundamental nature of a system, so also is the arrangements of the parts--that is,the system **"structure."** The gears, springs, and other parts of a watch interact to move the hands through minutes and hours only because they are all arranged in certain specified ways. Even the smallest change in the positioning of parts will result in the watch going slower or faster than desired, or perhaps not going at all.

Social Systems

Now consider **social systems**. They can also be said to be more than the sum of the individuals that compose them. Different patterns of interactions among people produce different kinds of systems. Forty young people in a room at a university, for example, might constitute a class. Depending on their interactions, however, they might also be a conspiracy, a party, a mob, an orgy, a club, or just forty separate individuals in a room. In each of these possibilities, the individuals are the same people: but if their interactions and purposes for interaction are different, the social system is different.

The existence of interaction and the rules for interacting combine individual components to form larger, interrelated wholes. "Gestalt" is a concept used to indicate this phenomenon of the whole being more than the sum of its parts. A social gestalt is formed from the individuals plus the sum total of their relationships. The character of the relationships is very important in differentiating different types of social groups or organizations from one another as composite or complex wholes, made up of interdependent parts. Thus, just as the structure and process in a watch, a car, a factory, or a hospital gives it its special character, so also the structure and process of a person or a human service system make it something more than just a cluster of individuals.

Change And Causation

By now you are probably becoming aware that social systems are always changing. Structures are only relatively permanent. All process implies movement; thus, social process, like all other processes, lead to change. This statement is based upon the fact that interactions between units in systems occur, and the fact that no interaction can be identically repeated because each successive interaction is a new experience preceded by the history of previous interactions. An old Chinese proverb states that, "No one can step into the same river twice," which is a way of explaining a principle of systems that--

"ALL SYSTEMS ARE DYNAMIC."

Movement, change, growth, corrosion, decay, and entropy, affect all aspects of our changing universe. Granted, some things seem to be more enduring than others, but eventually all things are affected by processes of change. Consider now that when we attempt to explain an event, or to relate why something happened, we are describing a system in which structure and process have been and are operating. Moreover, when we choose to describe or explain an event, in fact, we abstract certain **portions** of existence from the total space-time manifold much like taking a snapshot or looking at one frame on a motion-picture film.

A cartoon by Howard Post depicts two people, Alf and Sandy, who are shipwrecked on a desert isle. Sandy asks, "Why are we here Alf?" Alf replies, "Theologians might say we're here because he or (Heh-Heh) she willed it." "Scientists, on the other hand, say that we are an evolutionary stage of a protein molecule." "Politicians might say that we're here merely to be governed." "Why do you think we're here, Sandy?" Sandy quips, "I think we're here because you bought us a cheap boat and crummy charts."

The cartoon illustrates one of the main benefits of systems theory as well as one of its limitations; namely, that the systems approach tells us that we should recognize and interrelate many otherwise discrete bits of information, though it does not tell us which pieces are important or how to fit them together. The cartoon depicts a series of interactions between two people--a fairly short portion of an extended, complex reality. The dialogue causes you to focus on the question of how these two people came to be on the island.

Several explanations are put forward, but there is no indication of which is correct. In fact, a moment's reflection leads to the realization that neither one explanation nor any other is correct. Rather, each may be correct from a particular point of view, and perhaps even all are correct if we consider that each may explain selected aspects of the total "cause." Moreover, there are many other explanations--social, biological, meteorological, chemical, and psychological, for example--that could also contribute to a broader understanding of the situation.

It has already been mentioned that man's knowledge about the universe has mushroomed. At the same time, there has been a tendency toward specialization and division. Scholars (and others) typically seek to explain the world in terms of what is called an approach or discipline. Thus there are biological, sociological, physical, ethical, economic, ecological, chemical, religious, political, psychological, and no doubt many other types of "partial" explanations for events. And almost every human event can be "explained" by each approach. A closer look at each explanation, however, makes it clear that each seeks to explain only a portion of reality. In recent years, the limitations of disciplinary approaches have been widely recognized and have led to attempts to synthesize more interdisciplinary understandings of the world.

As scholars in each discipline try to understand aspects of the phenomena which they seek to explain, the relevance of other disciplines becomes clearer. With increasing frequency we see works on social psychology, biochemistry, political economy, sociobiology, cultural anthropology, and community ecology, to name a few. Each of these interdisciplinary approaches recognizes the interdependent nature of reality and the limitations of disciplinary approaches to knowledge. The systems approach takes this a step further by suggesting that all knowledge can ultimately be integrated to create more complete explanations of the dynamics of human existence.

Specialization, Interdependence And Human Service Systems

The human services share this tension between specialization and wholeness. People and communities are whole systems, but for purposes of analysis and organization we divide them into more mangeable parts. Thus, as knowledge is divided into disciplines, communities and human services are divided into different policy areas, institutions and programs. Each part, or subsystem, tends to focus on some aspect of human development. When physical health is a concern, we develop medical care policies and programs. Theories of psychological processes lead to a mental health system. Violators of community standards require a law enforcement and justice system. When the economy leads to problems, assistance and income maintenance programs are developed. And so on, to the point that today we have specialists, and associated subsystems, for practically every aspect of human existence.

>>A high school dropout is selling illicit drugs for a living. Is this an educational, economic, or law enforcement issue?

A young woman is despondent over the fact that her marriage appears to be breaking up just as she learns she is pregnant. She could not have the child and support herself at the same time. Is this a mental health, marital, medical, income maintenance, child welfare, or legal problem?

Many people are being evicted from an inner-city tenement which has been condemned as unfit for habitation. Is this an issue of landlord upkeep, housing standards, enforcement, family, economic, or social service?

What alternatives are available in your local community for such situations? To what extent would people have a choice? Or would the outcome be dictated by the circumstance of whoever became aware of the issue first?<<

We also have a countertrend. Like not being able to "see the forest for the trees," overspecialization focuses on the parts sometimes to the detriment of the whole. The functioning, or mal-functioning, of one part often affects others; for example, a mal-functioning economic system may have implications for law enforcement, mental health, health and family systems, among others. Thus, we are now beginning to consider human services as a broader field which seeks to address the whole person, whole communities, and the overall organization of human service subsystems therein.

Let us make it clear, though, that recognition of the limitations of discipline-bound studies and specialization does not lead us to reject the disciplines or the professions. Specialization provides more manageable pieces of knowledge for inquiry. It also provides, and continues to produce, the building blocks for a more complete structure of understanding and operations; but it can also inhibit the interrelation of many partial truths.

A Reality Perspective

If you are beginning to think that systems are so complex that understanding them is well-nigh impossible, just relax a bit. While the systems approach does make us face the fact that there are many, many parts to systems, and that numerous systems interact and affect each other, it also allows us to confront the reality of causal explanation in human terms.

We can describe the behavior or character of a system or subsystems without analyzing each little part . . . or sub-part . . . or sub-sub-part. For example, we can explain how a bulldozer should go about excavating a hole for a new housing complex without analyzing its parts: carburetor, pistons, chassis, and others. Similarly, we are not compelled to ask why the structure is being built, or whether it is a government program--although these may, in fact, all relate to the broader explanation of the excavation. Likewise, we can design a system in which physicians, nurses, X-ray and cardiac units interact with patients without delving into why the health personnel chose their professions, the functioning of their internal organs and systems, and why a particular community uses a medical care approach rather than acupuncture, faith healing, chiropractic, or magical chants. This brings us to the "boundary problem" and two additional principles of systems analysis:

A SYSTEMS EXPLANATION IS ALWAYS LIMITED TO A GIVEN LEVEL OF ANALYSIS AND TO TIME/SPACE BOUNDARIES ESTABLISHED BY THE OBSERVER; and,

OUR KNOWLEDGE IS ALWAYS PARTIAL, DEALING WITH BUT A PORTION OF A LARGER WHOLE.

In each of the above examples, the focus is on a portion of the larger time-space-analytic continuum. The intent is to explain or to examine a portion of a much larger reality. When we pursue such a "partial explanation," we are in effect saying, "Let's look at this event and the immediate events surrounding it. Everything else is peripheral, or outside, the problem (or system) at hand." The systems approach would say that the immediate event under consideration is the "system of analysis." Everything outside is environment; everything inside is subsystem or process.

A few pages ago, you were asked to consider a watch. Return to that example. What is the purpose of the watch? What are the boundaries of the system which is directed to this purpose? If you said the watch is a time-telling system, are the springs, gears, hands, and other parts adequate to the task? NO! It takes a person looking at the watch to "tell the time"--in fact, a person with a particular type and level of understanding of the concept of time, the nature of watches or clocks, numbers, and like matters. Thus, the boundaries of a time-telling system extend beyond the watch itself to include other elements. If, however, the concern is simply one of determining what makes the hands of the watch go around in a particular direction and at a specific rate, we might limit the boundaries of our inquiry and explanation to the watch case and its contents.

How do we make judgments which allow such distinctions to be made? Let's depart from the complexities and principles of systems thinking for a moment, and consider the basic elements of any system.

Modeling Systems: Basic Concepts

A system is pictured (modeled) most simply as a "black box" with arrows going in and out depicting two key concepts--input and output. (Figure 3.1)

Figure 3.1

Basic System Model

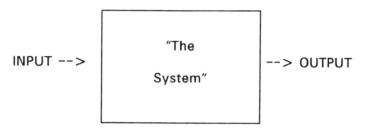

INPUT: That which goes into a system from its environment. A contribution or effect of the environment to the system under consideration.

OUTPUT: The action on, or contribution of, a system to its environment. That which comes from a system to its environment. The result of a system's action.

The conceptualization of a "basic system" shown in Figure 3.1 allows for the addition of other key systems concepts such as "conversion process." "environment," and "feedback." Each of these enhances our understanding of systems.

CONVERSION PROCESS: The series of activities or interactions within a system whereby inputs are transformed to produce outputs (e.g., steel comes into a factory from its environment; a conversion process takes place, and automobiles come out).

ENVIRONMENT: Everything outside of a system. The external conditions and influences which affect the operation, maintenance and change of a system.

FEEDBACK: The effect of the action of a system on itself. Information about a system's output which is communicated to the system.

Figure 3.2

Expanded Basic System Model

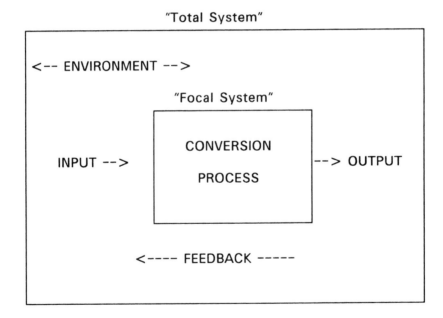

"Total System"

<-- ENVIRONMENT -->

"Focal System"

CONVERSION

PROCESS

INPUT -->

--> OUTPUT

<---- FEEDBACK -----

The result is the expanded system model in Figure 3.2 which both incorporates the latter concepts and raises questions about what "the system" is. Specifically, is "the system" the specific system of attention depicted by the inner box, or is it the totality of subsystems and environment depicted by the outer box? The "systems within systems" concept gives no answer to this question since it suggests that all are interrelated; but we cannot realistically or practically deal with the totality of all interactions in a community or the universe. Therefore, it is useful to adopt an analytic convention whereby we name the system of analysis (the inner box) the **"focal system,"** and the broader set of relationships is the **"total system."**

The expanded systems model thus places a system in its environmental context. **Inputs come from the environment, and outputs go to the environment. Feedback provides a new type of input in the form of information or effects from the environment about the system's actions (outputs).** For example, most people would picture the juvenile justice system as the process of taking inputs of delinquents from the community into "the system" of courts and institutions, and converting them into "outputs" of "normal" kids who are "rehabilitated." On their return to the community, information on how effectively the youngsters were rehabilitated is fed back into the system. This "feedback" of information on the quality of the conversion process has an effect on the future operation of the system. Such analyses are directed to understanding the dynamics of the **focal system**. If we expand our inquiry, however, and ask what environmental influences and subsystems affect the juvenile justice system, its relationships with other community subsystems, and the impact of the focal system's outputs on the community, we are dealing with a **total system** issue.

This approach raises questions about the nature and operation of systems, the relationships between subunits, and interactions with environmental systems. Several additional concepts facilitate consideration of systemic relationships.

INTERFACE: The point of contact of two or more systems or subsystems. The common boundary of two or more systems.

INTERACTION: Any process in which the action of one system causes an action by or change in another system. Reciprocal action between two systems. Contact between two systems, an interface, where the boundaries are penetrated thus linking them in a common event.

Note that inputs occur at the interface (point of contact) of the environment and a system and require interaction for the transfer to occur. Likewise, outputs require the system to effect an interface with the environment and to interact with environmental systems. Three concepts allow us to identify these relationships.

LINKAGE: A joining together or connection of systems or subsystems in a chain or series of interactions; e.g., communication, transportation, interdependent behaviors.

IMPACT: The effect or change in its environment, or environmental subsystems, brought about by the action (output) of a system.

OUTCOME: The end result, or effect, of an interactional process. The state of the broader system after an interaction or series of interactions between a system and its environment. Outcome generally involves changes in the environment (impact) **plus** changes in the acting system itself.

In recent years most of these concepts have come into use in daily conversation. (The word "feedback," interestingly, was not included in the 1963 edition of the Webster's Home University Dictionary.) These concepts provide a fundamental basis for developing a systematic approach to understanding a wide variety of phenomena in the real world. The next sections provide examples of the application of systems thinking in a several contexts.

An Ecological Example
Of Systems Thinking

The example of a fresh water cycle depicted below is a model of a system which functions to convert water into rain. The process modeled here involves a linkage of atoms of hydrogen and oxygen (water) located in a lake or sea in an environment of atmosphere and mountains. These elements are so structured to form a system that

Figure 3.3

The Fresh Water Cycle

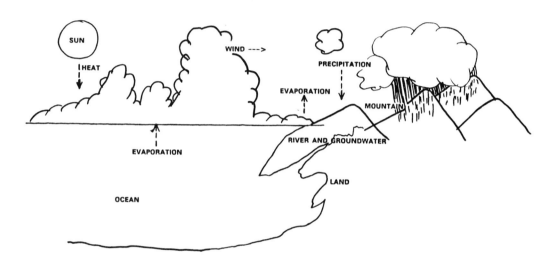

with the input of sunlight, (1) water evaporates, leading to (2) the rising of water vapor into the atmosphere to the point where, (3) cooling leads to (a) the formation of clouds, and (b) the circulation of warm moist air toward the mountains, which (4) causes the clouds to rise even higher, becoming cooler to the point of saturation because cool air is capable of retaining less water, thus (5) producing an output of rain. The rain then falls on the mountains and feeds back (6) to the sea. The entire process is then reiterated. (Each cycle of a system is called an "iteration". A system process which repeats is called an "iterative" process.)

In this **system** the **output** of rain may have **impact** on the mountains through erosion, and over time the **outcome** may be their flattening to the point that water vapor is lost by spillage or a channel is opened draining the lake. Note that this very simple explanation has used all of the systems concepts. Think of other explanations of simple events to illustrate your ability to use these concepts.

> >Try adding some further components to the water cycle model: (1) algae, fish, aquatic birds . . . (2) humans, industrialization . . .. Now, what are the outcome(s)?< <

Community And Social Systems

The systems approach can also be used to depict social systems and organizations such as human service systems, decisionmaking systems, and youth services systems. In the following models of these systems, try to identify the use of the various concepts.

A model of human services in a community is depicted in Figure 3.4 as the interaction of several community subsystems, each of which has the goal of helping people with problems. This systems model of community human services enables us to realize the limited scope of each of the community services subsystems in promoting human well-being. It also suggests that if human well-being is a goal, a linkage of many community subsystems may be required.

The introduction of the systems approach into the human services has led to recognition of the need for linkages and has generated a movement in several fields toward more integrated service delivery. Thus, health maintenance organizations (HMOs), community mental health programs, unified social service systems, area agencies for the aging, and multi-service centers are all popular directions in the human services today.

Figure 3.4

An Integrated Human Services System

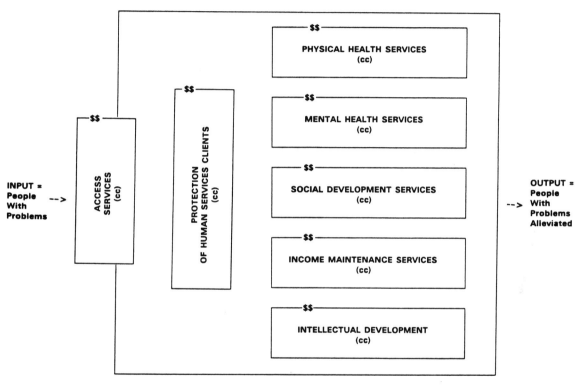

(cc) = Provision of Services
(Resource Expenditure on Client)

($$) = Delivery System Development and Support
(Resource expenditure to assure an
adequate, high-quality delivery system.)

Figure 3.5

Model of a Youth Services System

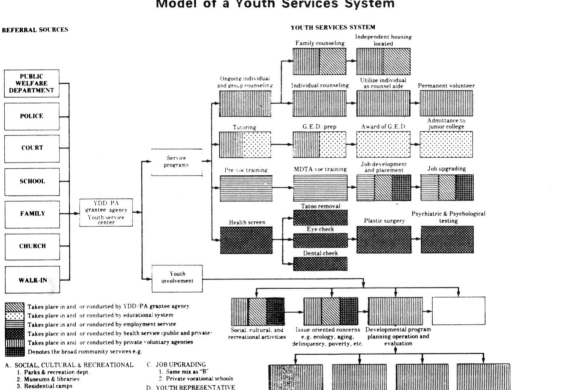

Source: U.S. DHEW, Office of Youth Development, "Challenge, Action, Change: A Community Guide for Youth Development (Undated, circa 1974).

In the area of juvenile justice, the service integration movement has stimulated the development of Youth Service Systems. In Figure 3.5 above, identify the sources of the "inputs." Would different referral sources tend to select different types of young people (e.g., truants, neglected children, unruly youngsters)?

What kinds of problems, even crimes, might each tend to overlook (or think of as being "none of their business")? What would it be like to be "processed" through this system? What "outputs" would you expect? How would friends and relatives tend to label and interact with these "outputs" in the future? What "impact" would this have on the young people involved? On the community? How might this system be different from a system of reform schools?

Community decisionmaking operations which formulate public policy, develop programs and enforce governmental actions can also be pictured as a system. The "political system" converts public demands for the allocation of community goods and services into governmental decisions and actions which establish public policy and carry out programs. (Figure 3.6) This model can be used to analyze practically any decisionmaking process, and will be used later as a basis for a model of the human service system.

The model indicates that inputs originate in the community from biological, ecological, personality and social subsystems which generate needs, expectations, opinions and desires of citizens. These effects from the environment create "wants" which are often presented to community authorities as requests (demands) for governmental action, and are the "inputs" to the political system. The nature of the conversion process, which may differ on local, state, and national levels--for example, the difference between the federal government with structured separation of powers, and many municipalities with a city manager system--then determines whether the demands will become inputs to the system, and how the ultimate decision will come out. (Easton, 1965)

The systems approach has shifted the attention of many political scientists from looking at strictly governmental actions to questioning why some demands get considered and others are excluded from consideration (called non-decisionmaking), as well as the more informal processes which affect the demand and conversion process. These same issues will prove useful in examining the functioning of human service systems. How are demands for specific human services generated? Why are some problems addressed by government and others are left to individuals or private agencies? Why are some rules enforced more vigorously than others? Why do some people get services, while others with similar problems are ignored?

Figure 3.6

Model of the Political System

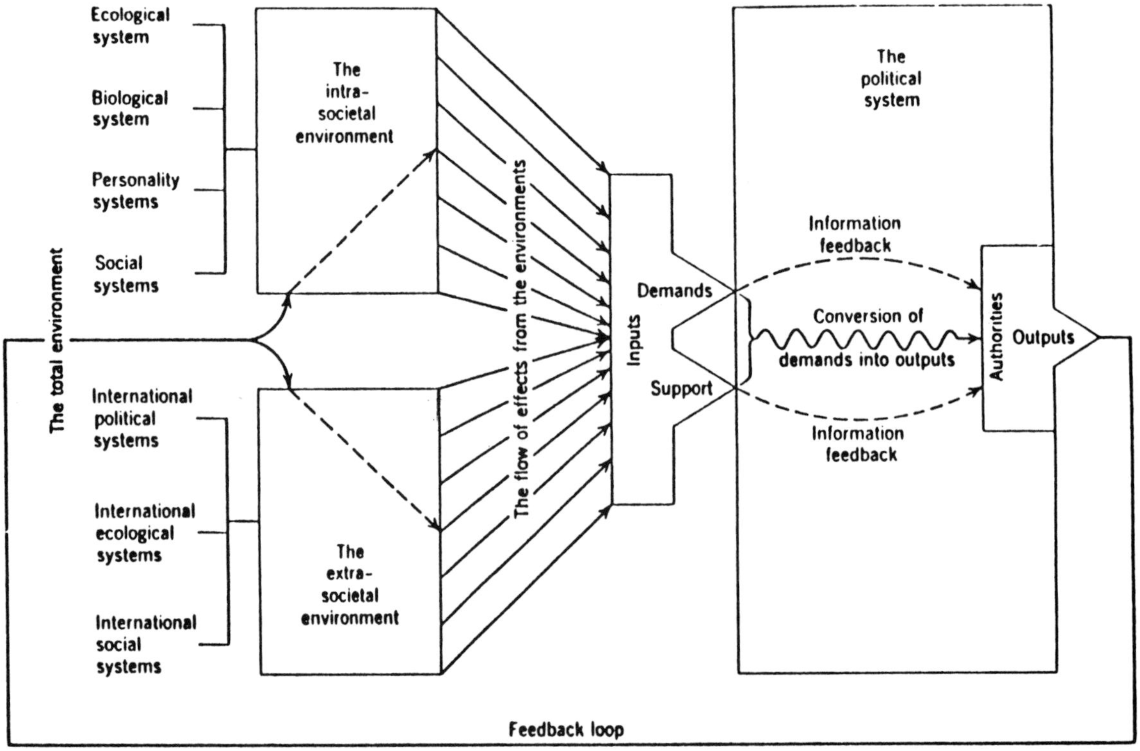

Source: David Easton. "Diagram 1," from, **A Systems Analysis of Political Life.** Chicago, IL.: University of Chicago Press.

A Demand Model Of Community Services

A simplified model of a community service system, pictured below, depicts a process which converts inputs of people and resources (taxes, staff, volunteers, and other contributions) by processing them through the institutions and agencies of the community and eventually returning the people to the community. The nature and amount of resources indicate specific levels of support for the system, and the nature and amount of people put into the system places demands on the resources of institutions and agencies. Together, in an interactional process, resources and demands determine the capability of the system to carry out its goals.

>>Create a model of the system you have chosen for your career, using this pattern. Identify the specific types of people--their needs or problems--resources, institutions, etc., for your system. <<

While this model depicts accurately many key processes of a human service system, it is far too simplistic for our purposes. First of all, it does not tell us how the people get selected for processing, or how some others are determined to be ineligible. What are the community referral sources actually like? What criteria are used to choose clients? What are the resources and how adequate are they? What is the ideology of the staff, the motivation of the volunteers, etc? What about the institutions and agencies--are they kind or harsh? Are they oriented to prevention, punishment, rehabilitation or custodial care? Do they seek to address the sources of problems, or is treatment directed to alleviating symptoms? Answers to questions like these are crucial to understanding (1) the interactional processes that occur in the community before certain people are selected out for treatment; (2) the interactional process that occurs at initial contact and at every point in the system; (3) the interactional process that continues after "output" returns the people to the community; and (4) the eventual outcome in terms of individual and community well-being.

The models of systems explored thus far utilize the "black box" concept of a system. Each focuses primarily on inputs and outputs which are fed back into the system. One objective of this book is to explain the character of several human service systems.

Figure 3.7

A Simplified Human Service System

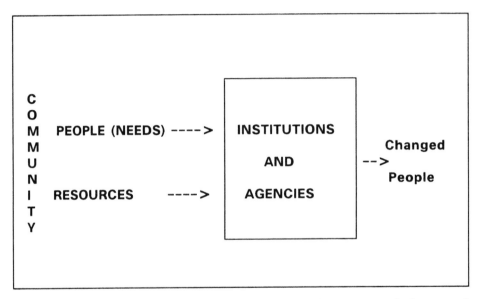

We wish to go further, however, and to enter the arena of change. It will be necessary, therefore, to look at the operation of systems, over time, in order to lend a dynamic aspect to our inquiry. And it will also be necessary to pry into the box and the little sub-boxes within to probe the interaction processes within the system and its subsystems, as well as between the system and its environment. The importance of the principles of systems thinking will become apparent as we examine the concept of community as a system in the next chapter, and in particular the role of human service systems in responding to human needs and problems.

Chapter III

REFERENCES

Beckett, John A. **Management Dynamics.** N. Y.: McGraw Hill, 1971.

Boulding, Kenneth E. **The Image.** Ann Arbor, Mich.: University of Michigan Press, 1966.

Churchman, C. West. **The Systems Approach.** N. Y.: Delacore Press, 1968.

Hall, A. D., and R. E. Fagen. "Definition of a System." **General Systems: Yearbook of the Society for the Advancement of General Systems Theory.** Vol. 1, pp. 18-28.

Lerner, Daniel, ed. **Cause and Effect.** N. Y.: The Free Press, 1965.

McIver, Robert M. **Social Causation.** N. Y.: Ginn and Co., 1942.

Optner, S.L. **Systems Analysis for Business Management.** 2nd Ed. Englewood Cliffs, N. J.: Prentice-Hall, Inc., 1968.

Post, Howard. **The Dropouts.** Philadelphia Inquirer, June 4, 1972.

Rapoport, Anatol. "General Systems Theory." **International Encyclopedia of the Social Sciences,** Vol. 15., p. 452.

Thompson, James D., and R. W. Hawkes. "Disaster, Community Organization and Administrative Process." In Zald and Rushing, **Organizations and Beyond: Selected Essays of James Thompson.** Lexington, Mass.: Lexington Books, 1976.

Von Bertalanffy, Ludwig. "Society for General Systems Research." **General Systems Yearbook.** Vol. 1, 1956, p. 1-10.

Webster's New World Dictionary. College Edition. N. Y.: The World Publishing Company, 1962.

Weiner, Norbert. **The Human Use of Human Beings.** Garden City, N. Y.: Doubleday & Co., 1954.

COMMUNITY SYSTEMS--Hyman and Miller

Chapter IV

COMMUNITY HUMAN SERVICE SYSTEMS

"The idea of the American community is deceptively simple, as long as one doesn't require a rigid definition."

–Roland Warren

Introduction

The preceding two chapters have dealt with the concepts of "policy" and "systems" in relation to social policies and human service systems in the United States. It was noted that social programs and human services delivery systems can be found in both the public (governmental) and the private (nongovernmental) sectors, and at all levels of society--national, state, and local. Among these levels, the local setting has a special significance for human services programs and delivery systems, for two important reasons.

First, the local community is the primary social context in which the human service needs of individuals and groups intersect with social policies and programs intended to help them meet these needs. As Warren notes, a principal function of the community as a social system is that it provides residents with local access to those activities and services necessary for daily living. (Warren, 1978, p. 9) This is not intended to mean that the underlying authority for or control of many of these services resides within the local community, for this is frequently not the case. Many locally based service systems, such as public schools, social welfare agencies, banks, and business corporations, may be dependent for their governing policies and operating methods on decisionmaking

113

authorities and headquarters staff in locations far beyond the community's boundaries. Nonetheless, the services these systems provide can still be regarded as "locality relevant," if they address the problems and meet the day-to-day needs of local residents.

It is also evident that local citizens, on their part, generally look first to service systems in their community locales when seeking help with problems of individual or group welfare. For example, the typical unemployed individual turns first to **local** sources of help in seeking a new job. This may involve the local office of the public employment service, private employment agencies, "walk-in" job applications to local employers, classified ads in local newspapers, and information about job openings received from relatives and friends. Similarly, the individual experiencing severe emotional stress may seek help from a local community mental health center or from a clinical psychologist in private practice, both local sources of help. A frail elderly person needing assistance with activities of daily living may request in-home services from a local home health agency to help in taking medicines and completing daily tasks of a personal and domestic nature.

As one moves to other problem-related areas of local community life, the same pattern prevails. A public child and youth services agency, though receiving the major share of its financial support from the state and federal governments, provides services to and, as necessary, arranges foster care locally for the neglected or abused child. Cases of alleged delinquency will be handled by a local court and juvenile authorities.

Not only is the local community an important arena in which to examine human services systems, there is hardly an area of local life that doesn't potentially fall within the scope of human services concern, either directly or indirectly. In fact, the local community can be legitimately looked upon as the principal setting in society for **delivery-level human services policy**. This takes into account both the services provided by formally organized public and private agencies, and other helping services available through informal sources, such as family, friends,and other mutual support groups. As we shall see later in this chapter, both formal and informal sources of help with human development problems are important constituent elements in the local community's human services system.

A second important reason for emphasizing the local community as a focal concern in contemporary human service systems is more pragmatic and political but, nonetheless, of great concern to local officials and professionals who plan, administer, and deliver human services. We are referring to the recent re-emergence of the local community as an important locus for planning and management in the human services arena. The current trend follows upon several decades of increasing centralization of authority and control over policies and programs at the level of the federal government. A signal event of this new shift towards decentralization of responsibility from the federal to local and state levels of government was the "new federalism" initiative, mentioned earlier in Chapter II. President Nixon clearly signalled his intent to push for this decentralization in his "State of the Union" message to Congress in 1971.

> The time has now come in America to reverse the flow of power and resources from the states and communities to Washington, and start power and resources flowing back . . . to the states and communities, and, more important, to the people all across America.

Magill has noted that the relationship of the federal government to the states and localities has been a continuing problematic issue since the nation's founding, having passed through several transitions. (Magill, 1979) However, since the advent of the Nixon "new federalism" initiative, the trend towards "returning power and decisionmaking authority in the area of domestic policy to the community level," has received continuing support from his presidential successors. (Magill, 1979, p. 101)

One of President Nixon's major achievements in this regard was the passage of the general revenue sharing legislation, enacted in 1972 as the "State and Local Fiscal Assistance Act." This was accompanied by other legislation utilizing block grants for particular domestic program purposes--for example, the Comprehensive Employment and Training Act (1973) and the Community Development Block Grant Program (1974)--and leaving considerable discretion to local and state government authorities as to how block-grant funds would be utilized locally within the general purposes of the authorizing legislation.

In the employment and training field, the more recent Jobs Partnership and Training Act of 1982, advocated and signed into law by President Reagan, offers an excellent example of a return to the traditional federalist philosophy of intergovernmental relationships in the American political system. The JTPA awards funds directly to the several states, leaving it to each state government to work out its relationships to local governments within its jurisdiction, and assigns to both the responsibility of arriving at publicly supported employment and training programs adapted to the varying needs of different states and localities.

Thus, from a political (and pragmatic) point of view, the local community, with all of its varied interest groups, ethnic compositions, and political persuasions, has received new emphasis as a focal point for decisionmaking and priority-setting in the planning and allocation of human services, at least in the public sector. But there is also parallel evidence that voluntary nonprofit human services organizations of national scope are also "tuning in" to this trend towards relocalization of responsibility.

This chapter focuses on the local community as an environment for the planning, management, and delivery of human services. The major topics covered include (1) the local community as an open social system, (2) vertical and horizontal patterns of relationships involving community systems and subsystems, (3) the nature of human services, (4) human services and human needs, and (5) a model of human service functions and resources in local settings.

The Local Community As A Social System

The concept of the local community as a **social system** is essential in understanding and interpreting the development and delivery of human services in the United States. In part, this stems from what Roland Warren (1978) has referred to as the "great change" in American communities. The local community's systemic connections to the larger society and its own internal structure have been altered dramatically in recent decades--toward greater interdependence, on the one hand, and more competition and confllict on the other. These changes have occurred under the influence of what Warren refers to as the three "master processes" affecting modern industrial societies--urbanization, industrialization, and bureaucratization. He depicts the effects of the "great change" in the following way:

> [The] 'great change' in community living includes the increasing orientation of local community units toward extracommunity systems of which they are a part, with a corresponding decline in community cohesion and autonomy. As the relation of community units to state and national systems strengthens, the locus of decisionmaking often shifts to places outside the community. . . . Thus, the ties between different local community units are weakened, and community autonomy, defined as control by local people over the establishment, goals, policies, and operations of local community units, is likewise reduced. (Warren, 1979, p. 52)

The decline of local community autonomy in relation to the larger society has posed for some the question whether the concept of community as a spatial locale continues to have relevance. Kaufman, for example, has noted that many regard the local community in an advanced urban-industrial society such as the United States as merely a "chunk of mass society," possessing little of importance that is distinctively indigenous. (Kaufman, 1959) According to this line of thought, most "local" activity is simply a reflection of institutions of the larger, mass society. (Stein, 1960)

While there can be little argument that the three "master processes" noted by Warren have altered the structures of local communities, a counterargument in favor of the continuing viability of the community concept can be made. (Hunter, 1975; Lee et al., 1984; Suttles, 1972) As we noted earlier, even those services and activities that are influenced and directly controlled by extra-community systems still possess locality relevance in the lives of a community's citizenry. And, as Bernard states in her defense of the community as a key spatial locale for most people, it remains the primary environment for their daily interactions, their experiences with problems of living, and their attempts to seek life satisfactions.

At the local community level there is confrontation, visual if not tactile, emotional if not intellectual. People still live next door to others, they eat, sleep, love, hate, avoid, or seek one another in a given locale. Whether or not they have much to do with their neighbors, they use the same grocery store or supermarket, attend the same movie houses, and patronize the same beauty parlors or barber shops. Owners or renters, they depend on the same community services such as, humble as they may be, garbage collection, street cleaning, and police protection. However emancipated the elite may be, it is still on the community scene that for most human beings interaction takes place. (Bernard, 1973, p. 187)

For our purposes in this chapter and elsewhere in the remainder of this book, we shall employ Warren's definition of the community in discussing local human services systems. He defines the community as **"that combination of social units and systems which perform the major functions having locality relevance."** (Warren, 1978, p. 9) In doing so, we fully accept the fact, as does Warren, that local communities and their various subsystems cannot be examined apart from their systemic relationships to larger social entities (suprasystems) such as state and federal governments and their various bureaucratic departments, and corporate headquarters in the domain of private organizations. It would be foolish, for example, to attempt to understand the operations of a local Headstart program for low-income, pre-school-age children without examining its relationship with the state and federal bureaus that supply its funding and stipulate certain policies for its operation. Similarly, a community's home health agency, though perhaps incorporated as a local nonprofit organization, is likely to be heavily dependent upon federal Medicare and Medicaid funds to support the majority of its services. In both instances, it is important to understand the agency's or program's relationships to other systems **within** the local area, and its relationships to systems **outside** the local environment. It is important to keep in mind the systems concepts from the preceding chapter, especially the system-within-systems principle and the system boundary issue, as we examine these varying types of systemic relationships in the next section.

Vertical and Horizontal Dimensions
Of Community Systems

Warren states that "In general systems terminology, one must conceptualize the community not as a closed system but as a highly open system with borders so permeable that they are difficult to define." (1978, p. 439) For our purposes, the question of the community's borders can be resolved operationally in a very practical, if not pragmatic, way. For human services in the public sector, we accept the relevant geographical area of the applicable local program's **jurisdiction** as establishing a meaningful local community context. In some instances, this will be coterminous with a municipal boundary, and in others a county or even multicounty area. Variations in these local system boundaries are often associated with differences in sectoral and/or jurisdictional policy mandates. For example, a juvenile or adult probation program may cover only a single county, while a community mental health service area may be multi-county in scope. Multi-county human service systems, often referred to as "joinders," are not uncommon when several adjoining counties are sparsely populated. In effect, these local settings are legally or administratively defined "service delivery areas" within the public human services sector. Similarly, most voluntary nonprofit human service agencies have defined geographic areas to which they limit their services--usually, a municipality or county. Proprietary human service organizations or programs sponsored by private businesses and industries may have less clearly delimited service areas, depending upon the geographic "market spread" in the one instance and, typically, upon the geographic locales of employees' residences in the other. However this may be, it is primarily the spatial boundaries constituting the local area for service delivery that we shall use in referring to "local" human services systems.

How, then, can relationships between human service systems **within** a local area be depicted, and how can relationships between the various systems and **extra-local systems be described?** For these purposes, Warren suggests differentiating between **horizontal** and **vertical** patterns of relationships in dealing with the question of the relation of community social-system units to other social systems. He defines the vertical pattern as "the structural and functional relations of its various social units and subsystems to extra-community systems." (Warren, 1978, p. 163) Correspondingly, the horizontal pattern is defined as "the structural and functional relation of its various social units and subsystems to each other." (1978, p. 164) No community system is completely uninfluenced by one or the other pattern, though there may be sizable differences among various systems in the local area with respect to the strength of their vertical articulation to extra-community systems or their horizontal articulation to other local systems.

For example, Duffee points out that correctional organizations may be situated within a local community area, but they are typically controlled and directed by remote bureaucratic departments of state government. In effect, they are "community-placed" service systems but not, in any real sense, "community-based" ones. (Duffee, 1980) Similarly, Tourigny and Miller found that various human service organizations in local communities differ considerably in the strength of their vertical and horizontal patterns. For example, some locally operated human service programs display a strong vertical articulation with extra-community sources of funding and regulations. Others have low degrees of vertical articulation but strong horizontal articulation in relationships with other local human service systems. (Tourigny and Miller, 1981; Tourigny, 1979). A typology of these differences, showing some of their implications for local policymaking and control of agency operations is shown in Table 4.1. In effect, then, the local community can be viewed as an **open social system** containing many subsystems having varying types of relationships among themselves (the horizontal pattern) and between themselves and extra-community sources of influence and control (the vertical pattern). In attempting to conceptualize community human services systems, the dimensions of vertical and horizontal patterns of relationships are critical considerations.

Human Services: Definitions And Functions

To this point, we have tended to use the label of "human services" as though it has a clear meaning among professionals and

Table 4.1

A Typology of Community-Based Agencies

VERTICAL ARTICULATION

HORIZONTAL ARTICULATION	STRONG	WEAK
STRONG	Policy established by local and extra-local units. Governing and/or advisory boards. Independent agency with partial dependence on on extra-local funding. Local and extra-local funding.	Policy established by local units only. Governing boards. Independent agency (may be affiliate of national association). Primarily local funding.
WEAK	Policy established by extra-local units. Advisory boards. Branch agency of larger extra-local system. Primarily extra-local funding.	Implicit policy. Informal leadership (made up of concerned citizens). Ad hoc or task force type organization. Insecure funding base.

Source: (Tourigny, 1979)

others identified with the planning, management, and delivery of services. This is not the case. Unfortunately, there is no clear consensus on what constitutes the boundaries of the "human services." This continues to be a topic of considerable discussion and some debate.

This section reviews some of the definitions that have been offered for the term "human services" and the types of functions these services are intended to fulfill in the lives of individuals and groups. Our purpose is to bring some order to the issue of definitions and to develop, for operational purposes in the remainder of this chapter, a useful framework for our discussion of **community** human service systems.

121

Morris has noted that arriving at a definition of the human services label is clouded by the fact that it has been and continues to be an evolving term within the general field of social welfare.

> The phrase 'human services' is the latest in a long history of phrases which seek to capture evolving conceptions about the well-being of individuals, the well-being of neighbors, and the well-being of communties. It is important--and realistic--to emphasize at the outset that discussions in this area have deep and often controversial roots in varying concepts of individual and collective responsibility for human well-being, and in differing perceptions of the social and political mechanisms to be used (or not to be used) in achieving or maintaining this status (Morris, 1977, p. 5).

Although, as Morris suggests, "human services" continues to be an evolving conception of organized responses to human needs, there is little question that the term is inextricably related to the concept of "social welfare." One can also find numerous definitions of this latter term. The following three definitions of "social welfare" are representative.

> 'Social welfare' is the organized system of social services and institutions, designed to aid individuals and groups to attain satisfying standards of life and health, and personal and social relationships which permit them to develop their full capacities and to promote their well-being in harmony with the needs of their families and community (Friedlander, 1955, p. 140).

> 'Social welfare' is an organized activity that aims at helping toward a mutual adjustment of individuals and their social environment. This objective is achieved through the use of techniques and methods which are designed to enable individuals, groups and communities to meet their needs and solve their problems of adjustment to a changing pattern of society, and through cooperative action to improve economic and social conditions (United Nations, 1959).

[T]hose formally organized and sponsored institutions, agencies and programs . . . which function to maintain or improve the economic conditions, health or interpersonal competence of some or all of a population. (Wilensky and Lebeaux, 1958, p. 17)

The foregoing definitions are sufficiently broad to cover the wide range of programs and services that fall under the general rubric of contemporary human services. As Morris notes, the human services can be viewed in a very narrow or broad way. In the narrow sense, "the term 'human services' is anchored to the idea of economic dependency, that is, in practice, to public assistance. The broader definition, however, "attempts to include as human services virtually all of the activities of modern society upon which the existence and well-being of citizens depend . . . ranging from the creation of jobs through the achievement and maintenance of a clean and pleasant environment to the production of conditions conducive to happiness." (Morris, 1977, p. 6) As will be seen in this chapter and throughout this book, we utilize the broader conceptualization, since it encompasses a diverse set of human development issues, not simply those involving people with welfare dependencies.

One important concern we have about the definitions of "social welfare" quoted above is that they primarily define the concept in terms of **formally organized** systems of services intended to meet the needs of individuals and collectivities. What is missing are references to **informal** sources of help, which are also important sources of human services in any community setting. These informal helping services include assistance received from relatives and friends, neighbors and neighborhood organizations, cooperatives, and many other mutual-aid resource networks that are indigenously organized and depend upon the voluntary help of individuals sharing a common interest, problem or need. As we shall see later, these nonprofessional, "lay" sources of help, along with many semiformal helping organizations, which we shall refer to as "quasi-institutional" systems, are important parts of a community's human services system.

Before moving on, let's summarize what has been suggested thus far about the human services label. First, the concept of "human services" overlaps definitions of "social welfare," and in many ways, the former is simply a reflection of the latter term. In contemporary usage, the human services label is likely to be less narrow in definition and more elaborate in practice. Second, human services concerns may direct attention to several different levels, or domains, of human need; for example, the individual, the family, neighborhood, community, or broader environment. Third, human services, like the social policies which give rise to them, are mechanisms of **intervention** for the well-being of individuals and groups, regardless of the level, or domain, at which the intervention is attempted. In sum, policies are interventions to establish the goals and objectives, and to specify the guidelines and mechanisms to be used in responding to human service needs. Human services, on the other hand, are the instruments of social policies, bringing helping services into direct encounter with both (1) the problem or need and (2) the recipient population toward which the policy aims are directed.

What types or specific forms of services fall under the general label of "human services"? To answer this question, it is necessary to explore some of the classifications that have been offered to sort out the different services by identifying "fields of service" or by specifying "service functions" in relation to human needs.

The Nominal Approach

Perhaps the most common approach to identifying what human services **are** is that which equates the label to a limited number of fields of service dealing with problems of individual and collective welfare. We refer to this as the "nominal" approach to arriving at a definition of human services. Sauber, for example, utilizes this approach in attempting to delimit the boundaries of the human services field.

The term 'human services' has proved confusing because it allows for multiple meanings and intepretations. For purposes of operational clarity, though, human services can be defined as including service delivery systems for mental health, social welfare, education, and criminal justice (Sauber, 1983, p. 16).

Sauber does go on to state that there are several other "overlapping service areas" that are frequently identified with the human services rubric, such as family planning, recreation, probation and parole, protective and foster care, vocational rehabilitation, and the like. In effect, though, Sauber, like many others in the field, simply accepts a limited set of broad "subsystems" dealing with an equally broad congeries of human development problems. In doing so, though, he is representative of many such general approaches relying on a few fields of services to define the boundaries of the label. Kammerman and Kahn (1976) also note that the label of "social services," which is nearly synonymous with that of human services, has traditionally focused attention on five fields of social welfare: education, health, income maintenance, housing, and employment. Harshbarger also uses a similar "fields of service" approach.

> [Human services] deal with those bio-social problems which arise from the vagaries and complexities of being human. Organizations which define themselves as in the fields of health, education, and welfare would, generally, fit this definition." (Harshbarger, 1974, p. 25)

Huttman views human services as the products of social policy aims. If, as she suggests, social policies are "plans of action and strategies for providing services," then it follows that those services falling under the rubric of social policy aims are, by definition, social (or human) services. These services she identifies as falling within the range of income maintenance, housing assistance, health and medical care, education programs, employment-related programs, and casework and group work services in the areas of counseling and community organization. (Huttman, 1981, pp. 5-7)

Macarov also notes that definitions of human services and social welfare typically rely on listings of **fields of service** (for example, services to families, children or the elderly, or services in psychiatric settings, health institutions, or correctional settings), or

types of services (for example, vocational rehabilitation, homemaker and home health services, family planning, job training and placement).

The "fields of service" or "types of services" approaches are not very satisfying ways of arriving at a clear definition of what human services **are** and what they are **for**. Followed to its conclusion, either approach ends up with an extensive "laundry list" of fields or types of services around which one assumes (or hopes?) a consensus exists among "human development professionals." Moreover, this **nominal** approach to a definition of human services provides few leads about the (1) types of human development needs that are presumably met by the myriad human services and the delivery systems providing them, or (2) ways in which coordination and integration among the different services and delivery systems might be achieved to the benefit of clients and to those making policy decisions about human services coordination and integration.

The Functional Approach

Another approach to delimiting the boundaries of the human services concept focuses on the various functions such services fulfill in relation to human needs. For example, Kahn (1973) distinguishes between the two categories of **"social utilities"** and **"case services."** According to Kahn, social utilities can be seen as analogous to other types of public communal services, such as a water supply, sewage system, postal system, public transportation, or highway network. These, he notes, are commonly accepted by the public as necessary parts of the infrastructure of industrial societies. Similarly, some human services are also widely accepted as constituting a "social infrastructure," though their forms and availability may vary from one locality to another. Such social utilities include public schools, parks, libraries, museums, public employment services, and information and access services. Their distinguishing characteristic within the social welfare field is that they exist for the common good and are available at user option (for example, libraries and museums) or by user status (for example, a community youth center and senior citizens centers). Many of these "social utility" forms of human services are supported directly by

126

public taxes and others by comparatively modest user charges (Kahn, 1973, pp. 77-78).

"Case services," Kahn's second functional category, are direct and tailored interventions into the lives of individuals or groups who are facing problems that are not resolvable on the basis of their own resources or through the utilization of the commonly available "social utilities." For example, the individual suffering mental stress, the married couple engaged in rancorous marital conflict, the abused child or spouse, or the juvenile gang engaging in delinquent acts illlustrate problems for which case services are designed to deal. Such services come into being as a result of individualized diagnosis and evaluation. Their general aim is to use a regimen of treatment services to restore or enhance an individual's or group's functioning in relation to particular needs as well as to community standards. (Kahn, 1973, p. 76)

> >Using Kahn's classification, list several other human services you would regard as "social utilities." Similarly, list several that you would regard as "case services." What criteria did you use to categorize a service into one class or the other?< <

Parihar (1984) also discusses human services in terms of their primary function of helping to maintain or enhance well-being and human development. He suggests that their functions can be viewed from both a **societal** and an **individual** level.

At the societal level, they perform three main functions: (1) socialization of the members of society into various future roles through such organizations as schools, training centers, and other educational institutions; (2) social control by identifying nonconforming members and by removing them, at least temporarily, from their role positions to allow the functioning of social institutions without serious disruptions, e.g., law enforcement agencies, mental health institutions, and correctional facilties; and (3) social integration by providing means and resources for resocialization such as counseling, rehabilitation, and related services to prevent social distintegration. At the individual level, human service organizations provide critical resources unavailable elsewhere such as education, medical services, and help with personal crises to enable people to improve, maintain, and restore their well-being. (Parihar, 1984, p. 3)

Hasenfeld and English refer to the human services in terms of the "people-changing" and "people-processing" techniques used by service-providing organizations. They note that "every person conducts transactions, voluntarily or involuntarily, with a whole range of organizations whose explicit purpose is to shape, change, and control his behavior as well as confirm or redefine his social and personal status." (Hasenfeld and English, 1974, p. 1) Thus, human services are implicitly defined in terms of the major functions performed by the service-providing system. For example, "people-changing" human services include those provided by treatment organizations whose major functional responsibilities on behalf of communities and the society are socialization (or resocialization) and social control. These organizations include educational institutions, guidance clinics, mental health centers, mental hospitals, community corrections agencies, and correctional institutions. (Vinter, 1965) Such socialization and treatment organizations and the services they provide are designed to "change people." This may variously involve services for educational development, resocialization into appropriate behavior patterns, or alterations of attitudes. The essential feature of this class of human services is that they intervene in the lives of clients to alter behavior or attitudinal patterns, thus enabling the individual or a group to deal more successfully with problems of daily living and to perform acceptable roles in community life. Vinter describes the ends sought by services provided through people-changing organizations in the following way.

A scope and permanence of change is customarily attempted that pervades the behavior of persons and endures beyond the period of their affiliation with the organization. People-changing organizations are usually concerned with effecting new and diffuse modes of behavior, new self-images or personalities--in sum, with altered persons in changed statuses. ((Vinter, 1965, p. 50)

"People-processing" services differ from "people-changing" services in that they are provided through organizations "whose explicit function is not to change the behavior of people directly but to process them and confer public statuses on them." (Hasenfeld, 1972, p. 256) Examples of people-processing services would involve such service delivery systems as (1) a diagnostic clinic, which **refers** individuals to other provider systems for direct services, (2) an employment placement office, which **links** the job seeker with a potential employers, (3) a juvenile court, which **decides** the disposition of an adjudged delinquent youth and mandates juvenile probation within the community or institutionalization, and (4) a university admissions office, which may **determine** those applicants accepted for admission and those rejected.

Hasenfeld depicts the functions of "people-processing" systems in the following way.

These organizations shape a person's life by controlling his access to a wide range of social settings through the public status they confer; and they may define and confirm the individual's social position when his current status is questioned (Hasenfeld, 1972, p. 256).

(Although it will be discussed later, we should also note here many informal, "lay" service systems within the local community perform "people-processing" functions. For example, many of us often turn to friends and acquaintances to help us decide whether to seek professional treatment for a physical or emotional ailment, and frequently rely on their recommendations of which practitioners within the local community are the "best" for a given condition or problem. These, too, are instances of "people-processing" services, although not provided by a recognized human services professional. The essence of people-processing is the classification and disposition of the individual in need of help, regardless of who the helping agent might be.)

In relation to problems associated with life-span human development processes, Urban and Vondracek present a threefold typology of community service systems, each performing a different function with respect to individuals and families--the two primary units of concern in their writing. They label these (1) **prime** community services systems; (2) **backup** community services systems; and (3) **informal helping networks**. (Urban and Vondracek, pp. 431 ff.)

Prime community service systems are similar to what Kahn (see above) refers to as "social utilities." They include those community-based service-providing systems that represent "the institutional context for fostering the development of individuals and families." (Urban and Vondracek, p. 431) Although communities may vary in their ability to provide these services, they typically include service systems dealing with public education, recreation, religion, public health, sanitation, transportation, housing, employment, and legal concerns.

Backup community service systems exist to deal with problems in human development that cannot be accommodated through the "prime" community systems. According to Urban and Vondracek, "The system of community backup services is concerned with promoting the constructive development of people and, therefore, is called the **human services system.**" (p. 431) Examples of community backup services are similar to what Kahn refers to as "case services" (see above) and what Vinter has called "treatment services" (see above).

The informal helping network, which constitutes the third community services system in Urban and Vondracek's conceptualization, is quite similar to what we earlier referred to as "lay" human services within local communities. As Urban and Vondracek note (and we heartily agree), many people prefer to rely on informal means for getting help with their problems, eschewing the formal human services systems unless absolutely necessary. Who are these informal, "lay" helpers? "Such care-givers may include the clergy, teachers, police, ambulance drivers, Sunday School teachers, volunteers, business people, bartenders, building superintendents, or simply neighborhood friends." (Urban and Vondracek, 1977, p. 432; also, see Gottlieb, 1976, on mutual help groups).

>>Using Urban and Vondracek's threefold classification, list several community service systems you would classify as prime systems, backup systems, or informal helping networks. What similarities and differences do you see between these three categories and some of those discussed earlier--from Kahn, Hasenfeld, and Vinter, for example?<<

Before ending this section on functional approaches, we wish to present one more scheme which is instructive on the nature of human services and human services programs. Morehouse (1970) developed a typology of social programs, based on his interest in designing appropriate ways of evaluating the several innovative programs associated with the Equal Opportunity Act of 1964 (popularly referred to as the "Anti-Poverty Act"). The typology essentially emerged from Morehouse's frustrations with efforts to evaluate the various anti-poverty programs, which differed greatly among themselves in form and character. Consequently, he developed a four-cell typology, based on two principal axes, each representing an important dimension of the programs. One principal axis of his typology divides services into two broad categories, based on the service program's aims and objectives: maintenance and opportunity. "A maintenance program is one that provides tangible goods and services." (1970, p. 100) Such goods and services might include, for example, cash assistance, food stamps, health care, and housing. These, of course, are the more obvious forms of maintenance services. If, by maintenance services, one is referring to services directed toward **direct** satisfaction of physical and material needs, other services aimed toward protection and individual security--for example, police patrol, foster and day care for children and elderly--could also be included.

Opportunity-producing services, on the other hand, are concerned with equipping individuals and groups with skills, education and the like, so that they can take advantage of future opportunities to sustain or improve their life styles and levels of living. As Morehouse notes:

> An opportunity program . . . is concerned not with directly meeting the materials needs of a [target] group, but with increasing the group's capabilities or opportunities to bring about a positive change in an individual's capacity to earn or to learn (Morehouse, 1970, p. 10).

Examples of opportunity-producing programs include job training services to equip a person to obtain new or better employment, adult education, compensatory education (such as Headstart), and professional technical assistance to neighborhood and other community groups. In effect, opportunity-producing services help individuals and groups to increase their capacity to compete successfully in everyday life. (We would add that opportunity-producing service programs may also be directed both towards rehabilitation--as in the sense of job training for new occupational lines, clinical counseling to deal with problems of lowered psychological functioning--or a community economic development program geared towards attracting new industry and jobs to the local area but not with **specific** job seekers in mind as potential employees.)

>>List a number of services you would regard as being (1) of a maintenance type or (2) of an opportunity-producing type. What criteria did you use to classify a service into one or the other of these categories?<<

The second dimension of Morehouse's typology also relates to the aims and objectives of the service program; principally, to their scope or breadth. The distinction he makes is between "specific-aim" and "broad-aim" programs, drawing upon earlier work by Weiss and Rein (1969). The former identifies services that can be precisely specified because they are directed towards a narrow area

132

of human need; for example, rent supplements, legal services, preventive medicine, and the like. They combine tangibility and a definite target population. Broad-aim services, on the other hand, are more concerned with more the multifaceted processes of development, such as citizen participation and involvement in community life, long-term economic development, or downtown revitalization. Certainly, these are not unimportant programs for local communities and their citizens, but their broad aims and processual features make them difficult to specify with respect to precise intervention targets and beneficiaries. Moreover, for many such programs, the benefits of the services provided may not become visible for some length of time, inasmuch as they are really directed, in many instances, toward modification and/or reform of existing institutional patterns in the community. In effect, Morehouse ends up with a four-cell typology of social programs, as shown in Figure 4.1 below.

Macarov has also suggested a classification of helping services not too unlike that of Morehouse. He suggests that helping services, or aid, given to individuals and groups may be categorized into one of three types:

> [The] aid may be direct, as is a financial grant; semidirect, as is training in work habits for successful job placement; or indirect, as is engaging in social action to have needs met through establishing a new agency or making changes either in existing ones or in society as a whole (Macarov, 1979, p. 25).

In this section, we have reviewed a number of approaches to defining and/or classifying "human services." How these various approaches fit together in providing the basis for understanding and interpreting the topography of human services at the local community level will be the subject of discussion in a later section. Before that, though, we wish to focus on another concern regarding human services that has not been explicitly dealt with heretofore. This is the concept of "need" in relation to the provision of human services. In short, what do we mean when we say that human services respond to the needs of individuals, families, or even entire communities? Or, stated in another way, what do we mean when we

Figure 4.1

Typology of Social Programs

Scope of Service Aims	Nature of Service Aims	
	Maintenance	Opportunity
Specific-Aim Objectives	TYPE I Specific-Aim/ Maintenance Services	TYPE II Specific-Aim/ Opportunity Services
Broad-Aim Objectives	TYPE III Broad-Aim/ Maintenance Services	TYPE IV Broad-Aim/ Opportunity Services

(Adapted from Morehouse, 1970)

state that the primary function of social policy is to provide a **collective** response to **personal** problems and needs? That is the focus of the next section.

Human Services
And Human Needs

As we have noted before, human services are forms of intervention, as are the social policies and programs from which they originate. As one moves down the hierarchy of concepts, from policy to program to services delivery, there is an increasing amount of specificity in immediate aims and targets, with the level of service delivery being the most specific. It is at the level of service delivery that policy and program objectives intersect with human needs, problems, and desires.

We should always remember, though, that programs and services only come into being when a need or problem is recognized. As Loewenberg and Dolgoff (1972) write:

> Social intervention generally occurs in reponse to someone identifying a condition as problematic or faulty . . . unless a condition becomes identified as a problem, it will not receive attention and will not become the objective of any social intervention activity. (p. 13)

Most of the physical, material and emotional needs of individuals and families are met without external professional help or, for that matter, informal sources of help. It is only when meeting a **need** becomes problematic to the individual, family, or community-- that is, when there is a discrepancy between what **is** and what **should be** in the area of human need--that intervention in the form of human services is called for. Whether such intervention actually occurs is, of course, problematic in and of itself. Not all human service needs receive attention. This is particularly the case in the United States, where requests for help rely mainly on the initiative of the individual or group in need to actively seek help. In some instances, there may a reluctance on the part of an individual to seek outside help, because of a fear of stigma or an abiding belief that one should handle one's own problems without outside help. In other cases, individuals may simply not be knowledgeable about the range of services available within the local area to assist with problems in human development. Unfortunately, in still other cases, the needed service may simply not be available locally, or eligibility criteria may exclude an individual from receiving help from a public human services agency. As Sauber suggests, meeting human service needs is a matter of linking systematically the client (service need or demand) and an available service program (service provision). (Sauber, 1983, pp. 13-15) Both are necesssary ingredients in forging the program-client system that is the essence of delivery in the human services.

What, then, constitutes human service needs? How can they be classified, in order to provide a basis for understanding and assessing community human service systems? To deal with this question, we shall draw upon a classification of needs offered by Macarov. He suggests a threefold classification:

o **Common human needs**

o **Special needs**

o **Societally caused needs**

The first category in Macarov's classification pertains to **common human needs**. He relates this category to Maslow's approach to human need (or, more correctly, to need satisfaction as the basis of human motivation). (Macarov, 1979, p. 25; Maslow, 1954) As Macarov notes regarding Maslow's hierarchy:

> In Maslow's formulation, the most basic needs are physiological, and until they achieve reasonable satisfaction, other needs are not felt. With satisfaction of the physiological needs, security needs become potent, followed by the need for love and the need for self-esteem. The highest, or final, level of need in Maslow's view is the need for self-actualization--the need to become everything one is capable of becoming, to use all of one's powers and abilities to the utmost (Macarov, 1979, pp. 25-26).

Macarov refers to the second category of human needs as **special needs**. He subdivides this category into five types of special needs, each referring to a different category of individuals. The **incapable** includes those who are unable to fend for themselves, because of physical and mental handicaps, the dependencies of childhood, or the frailties of old age. The **unprepared** includes those individuals or groups who, because of a lack of education, skills or necesssary social behaviors are not prepared for normal functioning in everyday life. The **disaster victims** include individuals and groups who are otherwise capable but have been assaulted by crises and catastrophes and are in need of at least temporary help to restore them to normal functioning. Such catastrophic circumstances may be the result of natural disasters (floods and earthquakes), environmental effects (air or water pollution), and civil disturbances such as riots. To these common types of disasters can be added other crises resulting from the death of a loved one, sudden loss of a job, or even the shock of sudden relocation to a new neighborhood or community. The **unconforming** include those who violate societal norms and are removed from everyday society or placed under formal controls while remaining in the community. This category, of course, encompasses juvenile delinquents, adult offenders, and others generally subsumed under the social heading of "deviant." The **unmotivated,** Macarov's last category, is one requiring further interpretation beyond its evident meaning. In sum, what constitutes lack of motivation may be a personal lack, but it also may be a response to continual rebuff in attempting to locate work or a loss of morale resulting from poor self-esteem. Whatever the case, though, there is little doubt that the category of the unmotivated plays a strong role in welfare policies and, currently, in the creation of "workfare" programs for welfare recipients regarded as unwilling to seek work on their own. It should also be noted that this category also extends to other areas of individual and group behavior; for example, the parents who do not provide adequate care to their children, or individuals who do not grasp educational opportunities as a means of personal advancement.

Macarov's third category of human needs he labels **societally caused needs.** Within this class of human needs fall such social concerns as ethnic and gender discrimination, structural unemployment resulting from broad-scaled industrial and technological changes, and changing economic conditions, such as inflation, that place pressures on individuals and families to sustain life styles and meet physical and material needs. (Macarov, 1979, pp. 26–28)

The importance of a human needs categorization such as Macarov's is that it calls our attention to the fact that human services and human welfare involve much more than simply dealing with problems of poverty, personal handicaps, and instances of temporary distress, however important these may be in the scheme of human welfare. It suggests that **human welfare and human development, as the principal concerns of the human services, encompass the entirety of a society's and a community's population**. Moreover, Macarov's category of "societally caused needs" should remind us that our penchant to locate problems in individuals and their personal deficiencies is a myopic viewpoint. For example, the current problems of displaced workers in the heavy manufacturing industries of steel and automobile production cannot be resolved by simply examining their personal characteristics or calling into question their motivation to work. Interventions at other levels are called for if problems of this sort are to be addressed; for example, policies and programs for economic growth, and large-scale training programs to equip displaced workers with new skills to meet the challenges of reindustrialization. In short, programmatic interventions must be targeted toward the **type** of need that is discovered, and appropriately focused on a **level** of intervention-- individual-, group-, or environmentally-oriented--that responds to the source of the problem.

A Typology of Community Human Services

The concepts and strands of thought from this and the preceding chapter can be combined to provide a typology of human service functions within local community environments and the different types of systems that provide these services. This typology deals with two principal concerns. First, it depicts major differences among providers of local human services (the vertical axis in Figure 4.2). Second, it portrays a range of different functions which human services fulfill within local community environments (the horizontal axis in Figure 4.2). As will be seen, we have mainly drawn upon the "functional," rather than the "nominal," approach in attempting to define and classify local human services and service providers (see the discussion above).

The general format of this typology is shown in Figure 4.2. Definitions and discussion of the component parts of the typology are presented in later sections.

We begin by addressing a question posed earlier in this chapter. What are human services? In general, we view human services as **help provided to individuals and groups in dealing with problems of physical, material, and emotional well-being, regardless of age, gender, income class, or locale**. Human services may be provided free of charge by tax-supported public agencies, by voluntary agencies supported by charitable and philanthropic contributions, by private practitioners and institutions through direct fee charges, or informally through networks of relatives, friends and mutual-support groups. In all instances, some form of intervention at the level of the individual, the group or neighborhood, the entire local community, or the general environment is presupposed by the very notion of human services.

If one goes beyond this very general definition of human services, a further breakdown into four main cagtegories of services can be made. First, many human service systems can be classified as **direct service** providers. This encompasses agencies and organizations, along with informal helping systems, that offer direct services to meet a defined problem of individual or collective welfare. Such services can be labeled **deficiency-meeting**. This may involve a tangible form of help, such as money, food, day care, homemaker service, health and medical care, protective services, and others which focus on immediate solutions to the presented problem or need. Other services within this category are similar to what Morehouse has referred to as **opportunity-producing** services. (Morehouse, 1970) These human services focus on providing help to individuals and groups by equipping them with new information, skills, or capabilities that enable them to take advantage of opportunities on their own. Services falling into this class include job training programs and some rehabilitative services, plus others, such as local economic development programs that focus on intervention at the community, rather than the individual or group, level.

A second major category of human services comprises what Hasenfeld (1972) has called **people-processing** services. These types of intermediary services are offered by agencies and organizations which use diagnostic tools and tests in attempting to match the individual or group in need with an appropriate helping service. For example, health screening programs, employment testing and job placement services, and diagnostic testing centers of many sorts fall within this category of human services. Additionally,

139

informal (or "lay") service systems often perform this people-processing function. Friedson, for example, has studied "lay referral structures" with respect to an individual's decision to seek professional help with human development problems. As shown in his research, lay referral processes often function as a bridge between the individual in need and professional helping systems. (Friedson, 1960)

A third category of human services is represented by **information-providing** systems, such as "911" emergency call numbers, "hot lines," local social service directories, local libraries, and information and referral centers that are often operated locally by a consortium of public and private human service agencies. This type of service differs from the people-processing services in that it only provides information and does not engage in diagnosis or testing before making information available.

The last category of human service system is comprised of the **policymaking, planning, administrative support, and advisory functions** that serve individual agencies or a range of agencies in the local community. For example, some general-purpose county and municipal governments have created departments of human services to perform planning and administrative oversight functions for all public human service agencies within their particular jurisdictions. In many instances, voluntary nonprofit agencies may also come together to support such mechanisms as community social planning councils and joint purchasing of equipment and supplies. Moreover, nearly all agencies, public and private, utilize advisory committees and task forces of local citizens to assist them in determining needs, planning service programs, and monitoring the results of programs. Although the systems in this final category do not directly offer services to client or consumer groups, they are important sources of assistance to the service-providing systems in the other three categories, through the provision of such supportive activities as planning, community education, grantsmanship, and fund-raising.

Figure 4.2
A Typology of Community Human Services

HUMAN SERVICE FUNCTIONS	SYSTEM LEVELS				
	Personal	Lay	Quasi-Institutional	Institutional	Inter-Organizational
Protective & Custodial					
Maintenance & Security					
Rehabilitative & Restorative					
Developmental & Enhancement					
Preventative & Institutional Modification					

System Levels: Organization and Resources

The general typology of community human services in Figure 4.2 depicts the interrelationship of the different levels of organization and resources (the horizontal axis) and the functions performed by human service systems (the vertical axis).

The horizontal axis in Figure 4.2 focuses our attention on the important issue of **who** provides human services in local community settings.* This dimension of the typology suggests, using Warren's terminology (1978), that there are various "locality-relevant" providers of human services within a community area. We can also view this from a general systems perspective by stating that the structure of **community** human services systems is comprised of many different **subsystems** which produce and deliver human services (output) to local citizens.

An essential aspect of the horizontal axis in Figure 4.2 is its suggestion that the range of local service-providing systems extends far beyond the traditional public agencies and voluntary nonprofit agencies that are usually the main topics of discussion in describing human service delivery systems at the community level (cf. Sauber, 1983). The typology presented here indicates that there is a continuum of helping sources--that is, human service providers-- within local community areas. They range from informally organized systems to those which are extensively and formally organized. All of these, we feel, properly fall within the domain of "human service provider."

Another way of looking at Figure 4.2 is to view each type of provider system as representing a particular sort of **resource** in the local community area. For example, established agencies ("institutional" systems) may have professional expertise and access to helping resources that simply are not available to individuals ("personal systems"), informal helpers ("lay systems"), or less established agencies and organizations ("quasi-institutional systems") in the community. On the other hand, informal (lay) sources of help

----

*   In part, the labels used in Figure 4.2 for the horizontal axis of the matrix were suggested by Donald Warren's studies of informal helping networks in urban communities (1980, 1981), though considerably modified as used here.

may be able to provide help more speedily **and,** at times, provide a better match between problem and solution than an established local agency. For example, in the area of job-seeking by the unemployed, there is considerable information from research studies to indicate that informal sources of job information--that is, friends, relatives, and acquaintances--are used more frequently and with greater success than are formal (institutional) sources of information about job openings.

Let's now move on to define more precisely and describe more clearly each of the types of human service provider systems shown on the horizontal axis in Figure 4.2.

The Personal Level

When personal problems arise and needs appear, many individuals choose to rely on their own resources, strengths, and capabilities to resolve problems concerning their own welfare. Although it may strike a discordant note in the ear of the trained human services professional, many individuals deliberately choose to deal personally with their problems without turning to outsiders for help. Personal solutions are frequently appropriate and successful, especially when the individual is insightful and well informed about her or his options. However, in other situations, personal solutions are often only partial resolutions of an underlying problem; that is, the individual's resolution of the problem may simply be "satisficing," although personally acceptable. (The concept of "satisficing" is taken from the work of Herbert Simon [1976], who noted that resolutions to decisionmaking problems are frequently made to "satisfy" and "suffice," given the current circumstances and knowledge of those making the decision. As Simon notes, we live in a world of "limited rationality," and to satisfice at the point of decisionmaking is more comfortable and less frustrating than is the search for an optimal solution.)

There are many other possible reasons why individuals may not turn to external sources of assistance in the local community as they deal with their problems. First, there may be attitudinal barriers toward having to rely on external help. Certainly, dominant societal values stress self-reliance and avoidance of dependence on outside

143

assistance, if at all possible, in dealing with one's material or emotional problems. Second, many individuals may be afraid that significant others--for example, relatives, friends, and co-workers-- will regard them as inadequate or unfit in some way if they seek external help for a problem. Third, a surprising number of people are often unaware of the various sources of help, formal and informal, available in their local communities to assist them in resolving problems. And fourth, some people simply have strong self- confidence in their ability to deal alone with problems of individual well-being.

One really doesn't have to search far to find illustrations of this personal level of human service resources. For example, many individuals turn to self-education for self-improvement through the use of books, do-it-yourself manuals, personal learning guides, and information in mass media publications as a source of development of self-confidence in being able to handle personal problems of everyday living. In other instances, the individual may take direct action on her/his own to confront others that may be associated with or even creating the problem; for example, complaining directly to public officials regarding the absence or poor state of public facilities, or negotiating directly with a boss or neighbor who is a source of personal harassment. Moreover, in cases of resource needs relating to money, food, and the like, many individuals simply decide to "go without" until things take a turn for the better. And, in many cases where the individual is suffering from too little income relative to personal needs and debt obligations, taking a second job to deal with the income shortfall is not at all a rare occurrence in local communities.

Generally speaking, we feel that the **personal** level of human service resouces has been too readily and easily overlooked when examining and assessing the local **human service system.** We grant that there is a lingering question of whether individuals who choose to rely on their own strengths and personal resources are making efficient decisions in relation to their problems. Nevertheless, this personal level is operative and it is extensive in local community settings. Regardless of an outside observer's feelings, it is a **real** option which many people choose and must be regarded as such.

>>What other examples of actions at the personal systems level can you list?<<

The Lay System Level

In every local community, regardless of size, one can find a number of informal help-giving networks existing alongside the professionally based human services organizations. These "lay" service systems are not staffed or administered in the same sense as formal agencies, they are not highly visible from the standpoint of having clearly established system boundaries, and they often go virtually unrecognized by those whose narrow professional training has led them to think of human service systems only in terms of agencies and organizations. But these lay service systems constitute important components of the total constellation of human service systems in the local community environment. They also have important roles to play in relation to local human service agencies, for they often make the difference for individuals with problems in deciding **whether** to seek professional help and **where** to seek this help. (Warren, 1980, 1981; D'Augelli et al., 1981; Caplan, 1964; Friedson, 1960; Kadushin, 1966; Gottlieb, 1976) As Donald Warren notes (1980), the lay service system often serves as an "invisible colleague" of the institutionalized human services system in local communities.

In the literature, the lay service system is referred to by many different names; for example, informal helping systems, helping networks, lay referral systems, informal support systems, and the like. For simplicity's sake, we have termed it here the "lay service system" level within the community's total human services system. In fact, it comprises several different types of informal human service subsystems at the community level. The average community resident will be a participant in many different sets of informal social relationships; for example, with relatives, friends, coworkers and acquaintances, among others. This may appear to make the concept of "lay service system" a bit overwhelming at first, but the basic idea is not at all that complex. Roland Warren has noted that such "mutual support" is one of the major functions of the community as a social system:

> Traditionally . . . mutual support, whether in the form of care in time of sickness, exchange of labor, or helping a local family in economic distress, has been performed locally very largely under such primary-group auspices as family and relatives, neighborhood groups, friendship groups, and local religious groups. (1978, p. 11)

Warren notes, however, that the influences of urbanization, industrialization, and bureaucratization have led to an increasing dependence on professionals employed by public and private service agencies and organizations. This erosion of the informal basis of mutual support in local communities is, in Warren's view, one of the products of the "great changes" altering the social structure of local communities and leading local citizens to rely more and more on the services of formal institutions in their daily lives. Thus, public schools assumed a growing number of functions traditionally performed within families, and social welfare agencies emerged as important sources of income assistance and counseling services. Nevertheless, lay service systems continue to exist with much greater influence and force than human service professionals often recognize or, perhaps, wish to recognize; they are an integral part of the local community's human service system.

Lay systems perform four important human service-related functions. First, they are important sources of assistance in helping the individual or group **define and clarify** what the problem is. Second, they are often sources of **direct help** to the individual or group--admittedly, nonprofessional in character but important, nonetheless. Third, they are frequently important agents of **referral** to other, professional sources of helping services in the local community. Fourth, they may serve as a rallying point for neighborhood residents and others with similar interests who wish to **organize and advocate** for particular changes in their local areas or in the community at large; for example, improved police patrols, enforcement of housing codes, and the like. Now, let's look more closely at each of these functions in order to understand more clearly what lay service systems are and what they do.

One important service provided by informal helping networks, or lay service systems, to individuals is that of helping to **define,**

sort out, and clarify what their problems are. This may involve simply lending a "sympathetic ear" or a much more intensive and mutual examination of the problems faced and instrumental ways in which solutions can be found. Both are important sources of initial help to the individual in need, but as Warren (1980) points out, a balanced mixture of the instrumental and the expressive is likely to be the most effective in helping the individual think through the problem systematically and assess alternative ways of dealing with it.

Research on natural helping networks, or lay service systems, indicates that the help-seeking process often starts long before the individual makes contact with an established human services agency. In fact, in many instances problems are resolved at the informal or lay level, and the client-agency contact is never established. In other cases, informal sources of help often supply the critical linkage between the potential client and the human services professional. Second, direct services provided through lay systems may involve a range of assistance given on an informal basis. The service providers typically include relatives, friends, neighbors, coworkers, and other acquaintances in the local community. All together, they constitute a "helping network" upon which the individual can draw in times of material, physical or emotional distress. Some examples of informal helping services avilable through lay systems include loans of money to individuals and families in order to "tide them over" until things get better, providing information about jobs to an unemployed worker, and, at times, simply lending a "sympathetic ear" to another's recounting of a problem.

At times, the lay system may itself organize informal services on a neighborhood or interest-group basis. For example, Collins (1973) writes of an informal day-care system organized on a neighborhood basis in Portland, Oregon, which was clearly effective in meeting the needs of residents without resort to formal day-care programs. In other instances, neighborhood residents have banded together to form "crime watch" programs for the mutual protection and security of homes and property. In many neighborhood settings, there is frequently a fair amount of "bartering" and exchanges of services among residents; for example, one individual repairing cracks in front walks in exchange for another tilling a vegetable garden. All of these illustrate lay systems or natural helping networks. Much more than is often realized, these lay services act as nonprofessional but effective responses to human needs.

Another area in which lay service systems have been found to be very helpful in complementing human services provided by professionals has been in after-care programs for individuals returned to the local community from mental health institutions or from prisons and juvenile corrections centers. These "community agents," as they are sometimes called, are often very instrumental in helping the recently released offender or returning mental health patient become readjusted to the everyday demands of community life. (Gottlieb, 1976, 1981; Warren, 1980; Caplan 1975)

A third important function of the lay service system is that of **referral** of individuals to formal human service agencies within the local community. This means that individuals with problems beyond their own capabilities for handling tend to seek the advice and assistance of friends, relatives and significant others before they seek professional help. These individuals comprise a "lay referral system," described by Friedson in the following statement.

> Indeed, the whole process of seeking help involves a network of potential consultants, from the intimate and informal confines of the nuclear family through successively more select, distant, and authoritative laymen, until the 'professional' is reached. This network of consultants, which is part of the local community and which impose form on the seeking of help, might be called the 'lay referral structure.' Taken together with the cultural understandings involved in the process, we may speak of it as the 'lay referral system.' (1960, p. 377)

What are typically called "self-referrals" to professional sources for help with human development problems occur in far fewer cases than many people realize. More often than not, the individual has talked over the problem with another "lay helper" first. This may be a spouse, other relative, friend, neighbor, coworker, or fellow church member, among others. It is likely that it is **because** the individual has been in touch with significant others who are "trusted" referral agents in her or his informal social networks that resort is initially taken to professional help with a problem. Such lay

148

referral agents may serve two important functions for the individual (or the group) in need of assistance about where to turn for help.

Lay systems may be instrumental in helping individuals overcome their fears of turning to external sources of professional help. Unfortunately, many human service professionals often do not realize how fearful a visit to an agency can be for some people. Helping individuals overcome their fears of being "overwhelmed" by the professional, helping them to realize that there is no stigma attached to seeking professional help, or simply helping them "come to terms" with the fact that professional attention is needed is an extremely important function fulfilled by lay helping networks.

In addition, lay referral agents may prevent individuals in need from being misinformed about sources of help available through community service agencies and organizations. There is considerable research evidence that relatively large numbers of local citizens are notoriously uninformed about specific sources of help available in their local communities for problems in human development. In short, the question of "Where can I go for help?" is a perplexing issue for many people. Lay referral agents are often important sources of reliable information about **where** to turn for help. (Sometimes, undoubtedly, they may also pass along poor information and thus impede the progress of the helping process.)

Many of the formal service agencies in communities have themselves attempted, in recent years, to deal more directly with citizens' lack of knowledge about potential sources of help with problems of individual or collective welfare. These attempts have essentially taken two forms. Many communities have established one-stop information and referral centers, available both to walk-in and telephone requests for information about human services have been developed in many local communities. However, it is not infrequent that many in the general citizenry have little knowledge that these "I and R" centers exist, much less the range of human services agencies they represent. There have also been a number of agency-initiated projects to train indigenous helpers to become more informed about locally available human services and thus to be more effective lay referral agents. (D'Augelli et al., 1981)

Virtually all of those who have studied and written about lay service systems emphasize the need for professionals to recognize both the authenticity of such systems as human service resources and the ways in which they may support and complement the professional's dealing with service users. Warren has forcefully stated the case with respect to those who enter treatment or therapy within mental health settings.

> In the vast majority of instances the therapy or treatment process itself relies for ultimate success on the role of informal helpers--families, friends, co-workers. The professional is always in an invisible partnership with a host of colleagues in the natural environment of the patient. The absence or subversion of the natural helpers is a major obstacle to treatment and often to diagnosis itself. (1980, p. 18)

A fourth major role which lay service systems may play in the lives of local citizens is that of providing a base of **organization for the advocacy** of particular interests or perceived needs. For example, neighbors may band together to call the attention of local officials to conditions they regard as problematic and in need of public response. These concerns may involve, for example, poor street lighting or lack of public playground facilities for children. These particular instances of lay system action are ones in which individuals may become involved both as action participants and as beneficiaries. They reflect a longstanding American tradition of self-help through indigenous community organization. Boorstin offers the following comment on this important American contribution to modern civilization.

> In Europe it was more usual for the voluntary actions of groups to grow up in the interstices of ancient government agencies. In America more often the collaborative activities of members of community were there first, and it was government that came into the interstices. Thus, while Americans acquired a wholesome respect for the force of the community organized into governments, they tended to feel toward it neither awe, nor reverence, nor terror. (Boorstin, in O'Connell, 1984, p. 132)

We have devoted a fair amount of space to a description of the lay system level of the community's human system. This is because we regard it as an extremely important component of the larger community system and one which is often overlooked in texts concerned with policies and programs in community human services.

We are not suggesting, though, that a reliance on lay sources of help with human development problems of an individual or group character is always effective. Both research and professional experience have shown that this is decidedly not true in all situations. Warren (1980), using data from a study of lay "helping networks" in the Detroit area, identified two important circumstances in which the lay helping system may not be successful in assisting individuals to find effective solutions to their problems.

First, lay help may be limited simply to "sympathetic listening" by a relative, friend, or acquaintance to another's problem. While possibly of some value in terms of emotional support, if the individual's problem at hand involves a tangible, life-sustaining need--such as a job after long-term unemployment, or information about how to apply for income maintenance help from a public welfare agency--then a sympathetic ear might not be very helpful, regardless of the immediate emotional sustenance it might provide. We do not mean by this to de-emphasize the supportive role another may be playing. But, in simple terms, the help being given is inadquate with respect to the **total** problem facing the individual in need. Warren refers to this as the "deficit pattern" of lay helping networks and describes it in the following way.

> As the problem load goes up or a life crisis situation emerges, the PAHN [problem anchored helping network] system may be limited in its capacity to prevent or 'treat' the emergent distress of the individual. No matter how sympathetic a spouse [or neighbor] may be to the need to find an effective employment role, or supportive of the desire of wife or husband to return to school, finding out how to apply and the early steps of coping with the new role may be beyond their experience, knowledge base, or understanding. (Warren, 1980, p. 11)

In the second case, the individual may engage in a kind of semirandom, "ransacking" behavior, seeking out so many possible helpers that the amount of advice and different points of view become so great that the seeker of help becomes confused and cannot make concrete decisions about how to confront the problem. Warren refers to this as the "complex pattern" within lay helping networks. In essence, the individual invests so much energy and time in seeking information, that the lay network becomes a "high cost system" resulting, quite possibly, in little payoff but much confusion. (Warren, 1980, pp. 11-13) According to Warren, the lay service system is most effective as a helping resource when there is a balance between expressive and instrumental responses to the individual's problems.

> The 'balanced' problem anchored network is one in which a sufficiently wide variety of helpers is accessible and used--primary, proximal or professional--and that like the pieces of a mosaic each offers a unique insight and distinct type of help tailored to the situation at hand. This rich tapestry of effective helping is one associated with the least stress. Both 'social support'--expressive reinforcement of the self--and active helping-- instrumental activities suggested by or actually initiated by one's PAHN [are involved]. (Warren, 1980, p. 13)

Having considered the first two levels in the community's human services system, we now move on to examine additional levels represented by organizations having varying degrees of formalization in their structures and operations.*

----

* We have not included a discussion of paraprofessionals in our treatment of lay service systems, though they are frequently regarded as indigenous, lay helpers in the human services. Most paraprofessionals, though, are employed as staff members by formal agencies and, as such, perform their work within institutionalized human service systems. Here, our interest is focused on lay service systems, which are typically not the human service systems in which paraprofessional workers are located.

>>What other examples of lay service systems can you identify, involving (1) problem definition, (2) direct services, (3) referrals, or (4) advocacy services?<<

The Quasi-Institutional Level

Many commentators on local human services distinguish only between informal helping relationships and networks (the "lay" systems level) and formal organizations (both public and private) that are commonly recognized as constituting the established human service agencies in the local community (the "institutional" level). We agree with Warren (1980, 1981) that there is a distinguishable category of local human service organizations intermediate to the lay and institutional levels. Warren refers to these organizations as "quasi-formal and "self-help systems." (1981, p. 18) We have designated this category as the "quasi-institutional" level.*

The quasi-institutional level of local human service systems and resources includes a variety of organizations that are responsive to particular and, at times, narrowly specific human service needs in the community. As a group, quasi-institutional human service organizations and programs have two key distinguishing features.

First, unlike lay service systems, they are formally organized operations, with identifiable structures of leadership, administration, and program goals. Many employ a small number of professional staff members, but in most cases it is likely that the bulk of the work will be carried out by volunteers and nonprofessional staff members.

Second, as compared to established human service agencies in the "institutional" category, quasi-institutional service systems typically fulfill one of three important functions: (1) provision of services that complement those available from the established

----

* The term "quasi" literally means "approximate" or "partial." The appropriateness of this designation is derived from the similarities and differences between organizations in this category and those in the "lay" and "institutional" categories.

agencies in the local community; (2) provision of services that supplement those available from the established agencies; and, (3) advocacy of change or reform in services or facilities available to local citizens.

We now move on to provide some illustrations of different types of quasi-institutional human service systems and resources that can be found in different local community settings. In doing so, we emphasize that our list is not in any sense exhaustive. The number and range of quasi-institutional systems in a particular community will vary with that community's characteristics; for example, population size, local values supporting the formation of nontraditional human service systems, and the variety of interests in the local community.* In general, though, it is possible to identify five major types of quasi-institutional human service systems: fledgling systems; self-help and mutual-aid groups; partial organizations; attached systems; and, temporary systems.

Fledgling Systems. Many human service organizations of the quasi-institutional type are comparatively young in relation to the established agencies in the local community. We refer to these as "fledgling systems." In many instances, organizations of this type came into being to meet a human services need that some individuals perceived as not being met--or, being met inadequately--by the established, professional agencies in the local setting. In this sense, many of these fledgling systems provide services which **supplement** those available from the institutional

----

* Roland Warren and associates (1974) developed the concept of "institutionalized thought structure" to explain why some types of new systems and innovative human service programs were accepted in certain local communities but not in others. This concept emerged from their comparative study of Model Cities programs in several local communities. In essence, they suggest that established social agencies in a community, which they label "community decision organizations" (CDOs), are prominent influences on the types of new systems or innovative programs that will be tolerated as part of the local human services network. A new human services organization that represents a strong challenge to the existing thought structure may engender intense opposition from the established CDOs.

human service agencies.

Fledgling human service organizations are, in effect, the "new kids on the block" relative to other credentialed and professionally staffed agencies in the community. In many instances, they originated from a coalescence of individuals sharing a common interest with respect to a perceived problem (or set of problems) in human development and an assessment that the problem area was being ignored or, at the least, inadequately accommodated by other agencies in the community. For example, many newly developed human service organizations directed towards the societal and community needs of women--sometimes called "Women's Resource Centers"--began as volunteer efforts to organize consciousness-raising and counseling activities to assist women with specific human development needs; for example, job improvement, spouse abuse, rape counseling, and the like. Gradually, many of these volunteer programs moved toward increased formalization of administration and operation, eventually becoming human service agencies, though still only marginally accepted as part of the local human services establishment.

Similarly, many crisis-intervention programs dealing with drug abuse began as low-budget, volunteer efforts to establish an array of crisis-oriented services unavailable either within or outside the mandate of the public children and youth agency in the community.

There are three outstanding features of what we have here referred to as "fledgling" human service systems of the quasi-institutional type. First, they tend to originate as efforts to fill perceived "gaps in service" provided by established human service agencies in the local community. Second, although many commence their operations as low-budget, sometimes storefront organizations, they tend to move towards the "institutional" systems category, or they go out of existence. Simply stated, it is extremely difficult to sustain the semiprofessional and volunteer basis of such an organization over time; budgetary pressures and human resource needs become consuming demands on those in charge of the organization. Third, many quasi-institutional systems of the fledgling variety tend to become more "professionally directed" with time. This, of course, is a concomitant of their movement towards increasing acceptance as part of the local "institutional" network of human services. As such, it is not uncommon for fledgling systems to begin to modify their original objective(s) of challenging the local human services "establishment" by gradually accepting and becoming part of the "institutionalized thought structure," to use Warren and associates' phraseology. (Warren et al., 1974)

>>What other examples of quasi-institutional, "fledgling" human service systems can you identify? What has been their history in sustaining their independent status relative to the "institutional" level of local human service systems? What do you feel their future will be; that is, do you think they will find it difficult to retain their independence, or do you think they have a fair chance of moving toward acceptance into the "institutional" network of local human services? What are the reasons for your conclusion?<<

Self-Help and Mutual-Aid Groups. A second important type of quasi-institutional human service system in local communities is represented by self-help and mutual-aid groups. Durman defines these organizations as "voluntary associations among individuals who share a common need or problem and who seek to use the group as a means of dealing with that need or problem." (1976, p. 433) Maguire notes that many of these groups developed from natural networks of friends who shared a mutual concern or problem. Their greater formalization of organization and operation clearly sets them apart from their original informal, or lay, origins.

[The] differences between self-help and mutual aid groups, as opposed to naturally developed networks consist primarily in the depth of formal organization rather than any more essential characteristics. In short, self-help groups are networks of people who consciously define membership, goals, and purposes, whereas most natural networks are groups of people with shifting memberships and no explicit or conscious purpose for acting. (Maguire, 1983, p. 83)

A variety of such organizations can be found in most local communities, each focused on a problem of special concern to a particular set of individuals or a group. In general, though, self-help and mutual-aid organizations can be classified into two subtypes.

First, many such organizations focus primarily on problems related to psychological, emotional, social, and physical needs of individuals. These include such organizations as Alcoholics Anonymous, Parents Anonymous, Reach for Recovery, Weight Watchers, and various women's consciousness-raising groups. Often, emphasis is placed on self-development or rehabilitation through personal efforts supported by other members of the mutual-aid organization.

In many instances, these organizations focus on problems that are also matters of public priority. Thus, in one sense they complement many services available through public human service agencies, and some projects of self-help organizations may be supported by financial grants from government agencies. However, as Borkman notes, it is often the element of "experiential knowledge"--that is, personal experience with the focal problem-- that distinguishes leadership and staffing patterns in self-help groups from professional agencies with a corresponding interest in the same problem area. (Borkman, 1976)

The second subtype of self-help and mutual-aid groups consists of locality-based associations that have a **communal**, rather than a self-expressive or rehabilitative emphasis. These include such voluntary associations as "food co-ops, block clubs, and similar groups in which the focal problem is not personal and emotional so much as concrete and communal." (Durman, 1976, p. 434) As such, they provide alternative channels for human services not ordinarily available through the established agencies in a community.

>>What other self-help and mutual-aid organizations can you name? What is each one's focus? How does it relate, if at all, to

other human service agencies in the local community?<<

Partial Human Service Organizations. There are a number of organizations in local communities that engage in help-giving activities, though their primary mission is not one of providing human services. We label these "partial" human service systems and place them in the quasi-institutional category of our typology. For example, many local service clubs, such as Kiwanis, Rotary International, Lions Clubs, Jaycees, Business and Professional Clubs, and the American Association of University Women, have both ongoing and special projects directed towards the needs of such community populations as young people, the elderly, low-income families, and individuals with special health problems. It is also not unusual for local business and industrial firms to become engaged in similar projects.

Many such projects are operated independently by the sponsoring organization, while others are conducted collaboratively with local agencies. For example, a number of community fund-raising campaigns, such as those of the United Way, American Heart Association, and American Cancer Society, are often spearheaded and cosponsored by local business organizations, working in partnership with representatives of social service and other community organizations.

The role of what we have here labeled "partial" systems as local human service agents is perhaps of greater importance than commonly recognized. This is particularly true as the decline in public funds for human services has highlighted the need for new types of collaboration among the public, private, and voluntary sectors in meeting human service needs at the local level.

>>List some other examples of "partial" systems in local communities? What services do they provide and for whom? How do they relate to other local human service agencies?<<

158

Attached Human Service Systems. We use the label of "attached" systems--as compared to "freestanding" agencies--to refer to human service operations that are located within such organizations as industrial corporations and labor unions. As Jorgensen notes, there are essentially three approaches to the delivery of workplace-sponsored social work services: "the social worker employed by the business or industry in a social service department, a human resource center, or a specifically titled department; the social worker employed by a labor union; and social work services delivered under private contract." (1981, p. 341) Social work services are, of course, only one type of industry-related human service. Health promotion programs, focusing both on primary prevention and direct intervention in relation to such problems as substance abuse, are also important workplace-related services. In fact, many social workers are part of the staff component in such programs.

> The staff for health promotion programs includes as many personnel types as the services and activities to be covered. Samples of professionals hired in such programs include health educator, exercise physiologist, counselor, social worker, mental health prevention professional, substance abuse counselor, and nutritionist. (Vicary and Resnick, 1982, p. 33)

Industrial- and union-related social services have a long, though somewhat checkered, history in the United States. This has ranged from early attempts by industry to enhance working conditions and productivity by "moral supervision" and the use of "welfare secretaries," to the use of industrial social workers during World War II, to the more recent development of "employee assistance programs" (EAPs) by many industrial firms. Many labor unions also have a long history of employing social workers and placing them in union offices or at union medical centers to serve the needs of their members. (Jorgensen, 1981)

Currently, there is a variety of human service programs attached to business and industrial organizations that can be classified under the general label of EAPs. These programs deal variously with a sizable number of employee-related problems; for example, drug and alcohol abuse, legal and financial problems, work stress and physical well-being, preparation for retirement, and family discord, among others. (Vicary and Resnik, 1982; Jorgensen, 1981) In recent years, the area of "career transition" programs designed to assist workers displaced by plant shutdowns and permanent layoffs has emerged as a critical human service concern in this "attached" systems area.

The extent of EAPs and other human service programs in business and industry is still not great, but those in existence are adjuncts to the established human services system in those communities where they exist. They serve to uncover and respond to a variety of human development problems that might not ordinarily come to the attention of local agencies until they had reached the point of serious deterioration.

>>Are there other examples of "attached" human service systems you can identify? What do you feel is the likely future of such service systems and programs; do you expect them to increase, remain about the same, or decline in number and extent?<<

Temporary Systems. There are a number of quasi-institutional human service organizations that are deliberately designed to be temporary operations. They come into being to serve a time-limited objective and go out of business when that objective is attained (or fails to be attained). We label these as "temporary" systems in the local human services field. For example, it is not unusual for such organizations to be formed to advocate a particular local reform or new facility relating to a human service need. This could be a land-use concern, with the organization formed to advocate changes in zoning regulations to permit construction or purchase of a group home for mentally retarded individuals. Or, it could be a temporary organization dedicated to **prevention** of zoning changes that would result in alterations to the perceived aesthetic quality of a neighborhood by construction of business establishments. Temporary organizations, as we are using the term here, seldom become involved in direct service-providing activities. More typically, they exist to push for particular changes their members see as influencing the quality of life in the local community environment. Their particular mission becomes the basis for both their formation and eventual dissolution. Some temporary organizations may make the transition to a new mission, once the original one is achieved, and thus become semipermanent operations. Most, however, have a limited life span.

>>What are some other examples of temporary human service systems? How do they relate to other local human service agencies? To local public officials?<<

As can be seen from the foregoing discussion, that labeled here the "quasi-institutional" level of local human service systems and resources encompasses a wide array of different types of organizations and services. With respect to the established, professionally based human service agencies in the community, they may offer services complementing, supplementing, or providing an alternative to those provided by the former. Whatever the particular case, they comprise a very important category of human service systems and resources at the local community level.

The Institutional Level

The institutional level of a community's human service systems and resources is comprised of those established agencies, both public and private, that have widespread (and often longstanding) acceptance and recognition--local, state, and national--as legitimate providers of local human services. For the most part, they are staffed by professionals and other trained specialists. Many of these agencies, especially those in the voluntary nonprofit sector, do utilize the services of unpaid volunteers, though on the whole to a lesser degree, proportionately, than organizations of the quasi-institutional type. Locally situated human service agencies in the institutional category can be classified into three general subtypes: public, voluntary nonprofit, and proprietary.

Public Agencies. Public human service agencies in the local community are financed directly by tax dollars and administered by some level of government--local, state, or federal. The majority of these agencies are mandated by law to provide a specified set of services to a particular segment of the local population. Traditionally, the service missions of the public agencies have focused primarily on nine broad areas of service: income transfer; education; health; mental health; juvenile justice; criminal justice; housing; employment and training; and personal social services.*

As we noted earlier in Chapter I, nearly all public human service agencies that operate in local community settings are enmeshed in some way in the intergovernmental system of relationships--either through financial support, regulatory control, administrative control, or perhaps all three. For example, in the majority of states, the local public assistance agency is actually a state-administered operation, though offices are situated in the local community. The same is true of the public employment service

----

*   In general, "personal social services" are adjuncts to several of the other human service areas listed above, but they tend to be more case-specific in character, responding to "unique needs and and institutional circumstances." (Kammerman and Kahn, 1977) Elsewhere, Kahn refers to personal (or general) social services in terms of "programs that protect or restore family life, help individuals cope with external or internalized problems, enhance development, and facilitate access through information, guidance, advocacy, concrete help of several kinds." (Kahn, 1973, p. 19) Mandell and Schram (1983) provide an extensive listing of what are commonly referred to as personal social services. Some examples from their listing include foster care and adoption, sheltered workshops for the handicapped and retarded, shelters for battered women and runaway teenagers, drug and alcohol programs, homemaker service and home health care for children, the elderly, and the handicapped, and protective services for abused and neglected children, among many others. (pp. 273-274) It should also be noted that personal human services are provided by all three types of agencies in the institutional systems category, well as many human service organizations of the quasi-institutional type.

office, which is a state agency with local outlets in various communities throughout a state. In fact, both of these programs involve relationships among all three levels of government--federal, state, and local.

In the case of public assistance programs--for example, Aid to Families with Dependent Children (AFDC)--federal dollars are made available to states on a matching basis, with the states accepting responsibility for administration of the AFDC program in compliance with federal regulations. State government, in turn, is responsible for the administration of the AFDC income-maintenance program through a series of local--usually, county-based--public welfare offices. For its part, the local community, in most instances involving county general-purpose government as the official body, has a role in the appointment of citizen's committees to serve in an advisory capacity to the local public assistance agency.

The public employment service, which was established by the federal Wagner-Peyser Act of 1933, is also an illustration of the intergovernmental system at work. Public employment agencies are financially supported by federal funds and administered by agencies of state government, but operate from branch offices in local community settings. Both the public employment service and public assistance agencies provide prime examples of established human service agencies that are "community-placed" but not truly "community-based" service systems. (Tourigny and Miller, 1981; Kaufman, 1959)

Many other public human service agencies in the local community are administered by local government--typically, county general-purpose government--though receiving financial support and subject to state and/or federal regulations. For example, in the State of Pennsylvania, Area Agencies on Aging, Children and Youth Services, Mental Health and Mental Retardation, and Drug and Alcohol Services are under the administrative control of County Commissioners, subject to regulations established by state government. On the other hand, Community Development Block Grants awarded to local communities of eligible population size primarily link municipal governments to the federal government, the latter principally through the federal Department of Housing and Urban Development.

The involvement of local public human service agencies in various intergovernmental relationships illustrates very clearly the character of the vertical patterns of relationships relating local community systems to extra-local social entities. Almost without exception, local public human service agencies have varying degrees of vertical articulation with extra-local systems through the web of statutory, funding, and regulatory mechanisms in the intergovernmental system. (Warren, 1978; Tourigny and Miller, 1981; Tourigny, 1979)

The public arena of human services in the United States has variously been referred to as a non-system, a mazeway of inpenetrable character, and a picket fence of interminable length-- each presenting an image of an incremental, piecemeal array of programs. In recent years, beginning with the "new federalism" of the Nixon administration and continuing into the 1980s, there have been deliberate attempts at the federal level to reduce the complexity of categorical human service programs by moving towards consolidated block grants for human services that would leave priority-setting and resource-allocating processes to states and localities. (Morris, 1977; Agranoff and Robins, 1982; Magill 1979) For example, the Omnibus Reconciliation Act of 1981, signed into law by President Reagan, consolidated nearly 30 special-purpose, federal categorical social programs into seven block grants to states and localities--although at reduced funding levels ranging from 20-25 percent for the various programs involved. Whether this "relocalization" of responsibility for public human services and movement towards block-grant funding, especially with the accompanying cutbacks in federal support, will result in greater effectiveness or efficiency in the local provision of public human services remains to be seen. Certainly, there is growing evidence that state governors and local government officials, themselves feeling the pressures of reduced state and local tax revenues, have not accepted the "new federalism" with equanimity. (Agranoff and Robins, 1982)

Voluntary Nonprofit Agencies. Voluntary nonprofit agencies comprise a second major component of the local community's set of institutional human service systems and resources. Voluntary agencies are of many different types, but at the institutional level, they are "essentially bureaucratic in structure, governed by an elected volunteer board of directors, employing professional or volunteer staff to provide a continuing social service to a clientele in the community." (Kramer, 1981, p. 9) Volunteer nonprofit agencies are private corporations, chartered by state governments to provide services on a not-for-profit basis.*

Local voluntary nonprofit agencies receive funding from varied sources. Recent estimates made by the Independent Sector indicate that nonprofit agencies in the social services sector received about 34 percent of their total income from governmental sources in 1981, with the remainder coming from contributions (30 percent), fees and charges (25 percent), and varied other sources--endowments, for example (11 percent). (Hodgkinson and Weitzman, 1984) Some of the voluntary agencies are highly dependent on governmental support obtained through purchase-of-service contracts and third-party reimbursements. For example, it is not unusual for a nonprofit home health agency to receive 80-90 percent of its total funds from governmental sources--principally Medicare and Medicaid.

Local voluntary nonprofit agencies also vary in their patterns of vertical and horizontal relationships with other systems. Some, such as local chapters of the American Heart Association, are vertically related to their parent state and national organizations, and their annual priorities reflect programmatic goals established at the state and national levels. Others, such as most home health agencies, family service agencies, and youth service bureaus, are essentially local in terms of their corporate standing, though perhaps very reliant on local, state and federal government programs for financial support.

----

* The not-for-profit basis of voluntary agencies does not mean that they cannot make a profit, only that any excess income cannot be distributed to owners or stockholders in the form of dividends. Most nonprofit agencies strive to carry over some retained earnings and contributed assets from year to year, as a means of protection against the exigencies of uncertain funding from one program period to the next. In recent years, as public funds for human services have been cut back and competition for private sources of funding has increased, this practice has become even more important for agencies of the voluntary nonprofit type.

Voluntary nonprofit agencies come in many sizes, from those employing only a few staff members to others employing several hundred. With the possible exception of income maintenance programs, they operate in all areas of the human services-- encompassing direct services, people-processing services, and social services planning.

Proprietary Agencies and Organizations. The third major component of the institutional level in the community's human service system consists of proprietary agencies and organizations offering human services on a for-profit basis. Proprietary human service systems combine a service mission with the commericial goal of generating profits for their owners or corporate stockholders. Although their entry into the human services field is still quite limited, they are increasingly found in the areas of nursing homes, day care, children's institutions, group homes, and home health.

Financial support for proprietary agencies is derived from both private and public sources. In the public arena, they also provide services through purchase-of-service contracts and third-party reimbursement programs similar to those negotiated with local and state governments by voluntary nonprofit agencies. As such, they are subject to the same policies and regulations in their provision of services to clients eligible for publicly supported human services. In size, proprietary service providers range from the single clinician or counselor in "private practice" to large corporations managing multiple institutions on an ownership, contract-fee, or performance-contracting basis.

The extent to which profit-making human service agencies will continue to increase their proportion of service provisions is, at this point, an open question. Kramer, for example, views the move towards reliance on profit-making agencies in the human services as a reflection of the "reprivatization" motif of current conservative trends characterizing many national and state governments. He notes that, "Reprivatization, or entrepreneurism, requires the use of the profit-making sector whenever possible and relies on competition in the market to deliver the best-quality service at the most reasonable price." (Kramer, 1981, p. 278) As might be expected, proprietary human service agencies have been the subject of intense criticism from many in the voluntary nonprofit sector. The criticisms have mainly been of two types: first, that human service goals and profit motives are not reconcilable; and second, that the profit aims of proprietary agencies lead them to focus on the "cream" of a particular clientele, leaving the more difficult and troublesome cases to the voluntary and public agencies. (Rubenstein et al., 1979) Whatever the merits of these criticisms, the evidence seems clear that the emerging role of proprietary agencies in selected areas of health, welfare, and educational services has presented the voluntary nonprofit agencies with a troublesome source of competition for clientele and for public financial support.

Prime and Backup Community Service Systems. The preceding sections identified the three major types of human service agencies constituting the institutional category of community human service systems. The institutional category can also be characterized in another way; namely, by the general types of community services provided through these agencies. For this purpose, we can refer to the work of Urban and Vondracek, who draw a distinction between "prime" and "backup" community service systems (1977).

Prime community services are the network of institutional services that exist in local communities for the development of individuals and groups, regardless of whether any of these are experiencing problems in human development.

The prime community services system can be viewed as representing the institutional context necessary for fostering the development of individuals and families. These resources are utilized independently of whether individuals or families have particular developmental problems. (Urban and Vondracek, 1977, p. 431)

They also note that the number and extent of prime services will vary among different communities, though usually included are such services as public education, recreation, religion, public health and safety, sanitation, transportation, communication, housing, employment, and legal services. To a great extent, Urban and Vondracek's concept of "prime community services" is very similar to Kahn's notion of "social utilities" in the meeting of common human development needs. (Kahn, 1973)

According to Urban and Vondracek, a community's **backup human services systems** come into play when problems in human development occur that cannot be helped through the normal operations of the prime service systems. For example, marital conflict, child neglect and abuse, strained emotions, juvenile delinquency, job displacement and long-term layoff, and physical decline of the elderly are examples of problems requiring deliberate interventions into the lives of individuals and groups facing them. "Indeed, problematic conditions may appear at any point throughout the life span, and these require specialized interventions and resources." (Urban and Vondracek, 1977, p. 431) Such interventions and the resources they require are the responsibility of the specialized service systems which constitute, in Urban and Vondracek's conceptualization, a community's "backup human services system." These services may be provided by any of the main types of agencies--public, voluntary nonprofit, or proprietary. In many instances--for example, protective services for the young and the elderly--public agencies may be mandated by law to see that services are delivered, though the actual provision of service may be carried out by a voluntary nonprofit or proprietary agency-- or, for that matter, by a human services organization of the quasi-institutional type--through contractual or other reimbursement arrangements with local or state government.

The Interorganizational Level

The interorganizational level of a community's human service system consists of the coordinated activities of two or more human service organizations that have combined their efforts, either voluntarily or by mandate of a higher authority, for a special purpose. Three types of interorganizational arrangements are of greatest interest here in developing a general profile of community human services and resources: (1) those focusing on policy development and planning; (2) those concerned with agency and program administration; and (3) those relating to coordinated services delivery.

Planning Functions. In recent years, principally in response to the "new federalism's" decentralization of priority-setting and planning responsibilities to states and localities, general-purpose local governments have begun to establish offices of human services planning. Typically, the responsibility of these units is to coordinate the program planning of all public human service agencies under the administrative control of the local government. Not infrequently, planning services are also extended to other local agencies in the private sector, since most of the latter provide some services through grants and contracts with one or more administering levels of government.

Private social planning organizations, supported by voluntary nonprofit agencies, United Way contributions, and outside grants and contracts, also exist in some larger metropolitan communities. Their primary functions are not dissimilar to those carried out by the human service planning offices in local government, except that the private organizations (sometimes call Health and Welfare Planning Councils) direct their efforts mainly to the interests of the private social agencies making up their constituency. In both instances, though, coordinated planning is viewed as a cost-effective mechanism that both serves the interests of individual agencies and identifies areas in which interagency collaboration can increase the overall effectiveness of the respective participants.

Administrative Functions. Interagency coordination through centralization of administrative functions is found primarily in the public sector, since the authority to establish such units and delegate them powers of administrative governance primarily resides in the public sector. Voluntary nonprofit agencies rely much more extensively on voluntaristic modes of interagency cooperation, since there is no supra-authority requiring one agency to cooperate with another.

Departments of Human Services or units with similar names are appearing more frequently as administrative units of local government. With human services consuming ever-increasing amounts of local government taxes and with the decline of state and federal support for human services, local government officials have moved, although quite gradually in most instances, towards better management and administrative control of the human service agencies under their jurisdiction. The result has been the creation of local departments of human services, with varying degrees of administrative control, depending upon the intents, if not the whims, of local government officials. In some instances, the central administrative unit may have extensive managerial authority delegated to it. In many others, likely the great majority of cases, the mandate will be more that of administrative coordination, rather than direct management control.

Service Delivery Functions. Interagency coordination at the point of service delivery has long been an ideal in the field of social welfare and human services. For the most part, though, reality has fallen far short of the ideal. (Perlman, 1975) Over the past two decades, there have been numerous experiments and demonstration projects concerned with coordinated services delivery in the human services. (Agranoff and Pattakos, 1979; March, 1968; U. S. Dept. of HEW, 1972) Essentially, these efforts can be boiled down to four general models of coordination.

The first model is reflected in co-sponsorship of information and referral centers by public and private community agencies. The major purpose of these centers is to improve the potential client's efficiency in learning about and getting in touch with the most appropriate human service agencies and resources to deal with a problem (or problems).

The second model moves one step upward from the first, adding diagnostic and testing services to the referral function. In this instance, both the efficiency of the potential client and of the potential service provider is enhanced.

The third model is frequently labeled the "case management" approach. Essentially, a single individual, the "case manager," works with the client from entry to exit, making certain that multiple services brought to bear on problems are coordinated and that continuity of services is sustained throughout the client's career in the human service system.

The fourth model is that of the multiservice center, which brings together the services of several different agencies in one physical location. The purpose of the multiservice center is to provide the individual or family with single-point entry to a range of helping services under one roof. The multiservice center is a popular approach to services coordination, although experiences have shown that it is a very difficult system to sustain over any period of time, given the proclivities of agencies and individual professionals to engage in "turf" protection.

Summary

The preceding discussion has focused on the different types of human service systems and resources that may be brought to bear on human development problems at the local community level. It was shown that a community's overall complex of human service providers is comprised of a diverse array of informal and formal networks and organizations. In the next section, we turn our attention to the major types of community service functions these various systems are intended to fulfill.

Community Human Service Functions

The preceding section focused on the issue of structure: **who** provides human services to individuals and groups at the local community level. In this section, we turn our attention to the vertical axis in Figure 4.2 and address the related question of function: **what** types of human services are provided in local community contexts. It is the interrelation of the **who** and the **what** issues that direct us to a conceptualization of human services as forms of human development intervention.

All human services, regardless of the particular service system involved or the specific help provided, are mechanisms of intervention. Their general aim is to assist individuals and groups in dealing with problems of human development. There are two important dimensions of human services as interventions that should be held in mind.

The first is the **temporal** dimension underlying the intervention and the helping services provided. For example, some human services may be crisis-oriented, as would be the case in instances of child abuse, battered spouses, threatened suicide, or drug overdose. For problems such as these, human services are directed toward a need requiring immediate and rapid response. In other cases, human services may be provided on a longer-term, continuing basis until a problem is resolved or external assistance is no longer required. For example, unemployment compensation until a new job is found, public assistance for low-income families with dependent-age children, and homemaker-home health services to assist a household member recuperating from surgery are illustrations of needs for longer-term human services that can eventually be terminated. In some instances, though, involving severe physical or mental disabilities, human service interventions may essentially be lifelong interventions aimed toward enabling individuals to maintain a reasonable level of security in everyday life.

The second important dimension of human services intervention pertains to the **target level,** or **social domain,** towards which an interventive activity is directed. Many human servces, especially those concerned with rehabilitative, therapeutic, and medical services, may be directed toward the **individual** as the interventive target. Other services may be oriented toward a **group** or **organization** as the object of intervention. This would be true, for example, in the case of services directed to families or to other population aggregates in the local community, such as youth, the elderly, neighborhood organizations, and the like. Health education and nutrition education programs, both of which have a prevention motive, also focus attention on the the needs of particular groups or target populations in the local community. Human services may also be oriented toward altering conditions in the local community's **environmental** context. Pollution control and local programs for economic and industrial development are both examples of environmentally oriented human development interventions, the former concerned with preventing environmental deterioration, and the latter with improving (or expanding) job opportunities and the locality's economic base.

Both of these dimensions of human service interventions, temporality and social domain, are important in understanding community human service functions and how they they meet the individual and collective needs of residents. (Loewenberg and Dolgoff, 1972; Urban and Vondracek, 1977; Mandell and Schram, 1983)

As we move on to discuss the community human service functions listed on the vertical axis in Figure 4.2, it is not our aim to provide an exhaustive listing of specific forms of locally provided human services. That would be an impossible task. As noted in earlier parts of this chapter, the concept of human services encompasses a diverse range of formal and informal types of aid, and to attempt to describe them in extensive detail would be a fruitless task. Moreover, there are sizable differences among localities in the types and range of available human services. This is attributable to such factors as population size of the local area, urban or rural locale, local sentiments toward the notion of "welfare," and priorities set for the use of a community's resources by its leadership.*

Our use of the systems perspective on local communities and their organization leads us to approach the **what** issue by describing community human services in terms of the functional contributions they make to the material, physical, and emotional well-being of individuals and groups. This means that the totality of a community's human service systems, both formal and informal, exists for the personal and collective welfare of its citizens. Even though many of the services, or financial support for them, originate from extra-local sources, the fact that they are **delivered** within the community makes them "locality relevant," regardless of their auspice or the patterns of vertical and horizontal relationships involved in their organization and delivery. (Warren, 1978) Local citizens have many expectations toward their communities and the life-sustaining functions available through its various service systems and facilities. Human services constitute one such expected community function.

Our approach, then, is to view a community's human services, regardless of the specific provider system(s) or particular service objective(s), as a set of welfare functions having locality relevance for the human development needs of local residents. As shown on the vertical axis in Figure 4.2 above, we have identified five general human service functions performed by the various levels of systems and resources found in different local community contexts. In the remainder of this section, each of these functional categories will be described and some illustrations offered of the various types of services and provider systems that come into play to meet different

----

* Interested readers may, however, find it useful to consult two of the references listed at the end of this chapter. Each contains detailed descriptions of a range of social services in the United States. These are Gilbert and Specht (1981), and Kammerman and Kahn (1977).

human development problems.

The Protective and Custodial Function

The protective and custodial function of community human services has two underlying purposes: first, **the protection of individuals and groups from harm or injury resulting from the acts of others** and second, **the protection of individuals and groups from harm or injury attributable to their own actions.**

For example, in the area of child welfare, protection of children against parental abuse has long been a concern. Through the doctrine of "parens patriae"--the state as the higher parent-- agencies of state government exercise their authority to intervene when parental responsibilities are not being carried out properly. The purpose of this intervention is to assure the protection and welfare of the child and, if deemed necessary, place the child under custodial care through removal from the home and placement in a foster family setting. It is possible that some lay service systems come into play with respect to child welfare--for example, a relative, neighbor or friend counseling a parent about abusive behavior towards a child--but if abuse or neglect continues, official action by the public child and youth services agency will be required to initiate protective and custodial care services.

There are many other examples to draw upon in illustrating the protective and custodial function of community human services. For example, crisis intervention services for rape victims, battered spouses, and drug-overdosed individuals may be provided by several different local human service organizations. Some of these provider systems will be established public or private social agencies, but what we earlier labeled the "quasi-institutional" service systems are also prominently represented in the crisis intervention area.

Individuals suffering from severe physical and mental handicaps, as well as the "frail elderly," may require helping services designed to protect them from inadvertent personal injury or harm. For example, home health agencies, which may be proprietary or voluntary nonprofit organizations, deliver homemaker, chore, and visiting nurse services to individuals whose physical conditions do not permit them to take care of their daily needs without threat of physical harm. In many instances, also, some of these needs may be taken care of by informal networks of neighbors and friends, who assist the physically or mentally impaired individual to deal with everyday personal needs.

Moving from the individual to the group level, we can also point to instances in which lay service networks are the mechanisms for the provision of protective services. In many communities, local neighborhood groups, often with the consultation and assistance of the local police department, have created "neighborhood crime watch" organizations as a means of mutual protection against personal assault and property destruction. These can be considered lay service systems, consisting of informal networks of neighborhood families who agree to "look out for one another" and responding to a particular protective need within the community.

Finally, we would also point out that the human services connected to a community's juvenile and criminal justice systems are partly directed towards the protective and custodial function. This may involve removing the law-violating individual from the everyday life of the community, through incarceration, or placing the adjudicated delinquent or adult criminal under the custodial watchcare of the community's probation system.

>>What other instances of community human services of the protective and custodial type can you identify? With respect to each one, what service systems, formal or informal, are typical providers of the service?<<

The Maintenance and Security Function

The primary purpose of the maintenance and security function of community human services is **to assist individuals and families in gaining access to resources enabling them to meet their daily material, physical, and social needs**. There are numerous concrete examples of human services created to respond to this community services function.

For example, the various income maintenance programs, of both the social insurance and public assistance types, are directed toward needs in this area. The social security retirement income program and public assistance programs for low-income elderly and families with dependent age children--the former a federal program, and the latter involving federal, state, and local governmments-- serve as illustrations. Additionally, there are income replacement (unemployment compensation) programs for the unemployed to sustain them financially until a new job is found. These programs are operated by state government through branch offices in various localities; moreover, these same branch offices house the public employment service, which can serve as a source of information about available jobs in the local community or in other geographic areas.

Publicly subsidized housing for the elderly of limited means and other low-income households, and public nutrition programs for the elderly also fall within this functional category of community human services, as does nursing home care for elderly individuals who can no longer take care of their daily needs without external helping services.

The above examples, of course, only touch the surface of community human services that supply help pertaining to the maintenance and security function. For example, lay service systems frequently provide temporary forms of help to individuals in economic distress; additionally, such systems may also be instrumental in helping the unemployed individual find a new job or in meeting the needs for social contact and companionship for the home-bound elderly or disabled person.

>>What other examples of human services responding to maintenance and security needs can be given? In each case, what is the objective of the service and what local providers of human services are able to meet the identified need?<<

The Rehabilitative and Restorative Function

The rehabilitative and restorative function of community human services has two related purposes: first, **to alter an existing dysfunctional condition of an individual or group** and second, **to restore the individual or group to economic and/or social statuses enabling them to live as normally as possible on a day-to-day basis in the community**. There are many examples of human services responding to this area of functional need, but we shall only point out a few as illustrations.

Counseling services for marital problems are available from a variety of established and quasi-institutional systems in the local community. Similarly, community mental health programs and services of private clinicians are available to assist individuals with problems of mental stress preventing them from functioning normally at work, in the home, or elsewhere in the community. Furthermore, as mentioned earlier in this chapter, many business and industrial firms have created employee assistance programs to aid workers (and sometimes other family members) with problems requiring rehabilitative measures, such as alcholism and substance abuse.

Job training programs for individuals with poor job skills and retraining programs for workers displaced from jobs because of plant closures or employee cutbacks also fall within this category of community human service functions. Similarly, vocational rehabilitation programs for the physically and mentally handicapped, in addition to providing health services and prosthetic devices, offer training-related services in skills centers and sheltered workshops as a means of improving the employability of their program participants.

The rehabilitative and restorative category of community human service functions encompasses an enormous and diverse array of specific services. It is also the area in which the interventive activity involving the professional and client is most intense among the several functional categories of human service.

>>What are some additional examples of human services of a rehabilitative and restorative type that can be identified in relation to

local communities? To what extent are lay and quasi-institutional service systems also involved in this area, along with the established public and private agencies?<<

The Developmental and Enhancement Function

The primary purpose of the developmental and enhancement function of community human services is **to help individuals and groups to maximize their development with respect to material, physical, or emotional well-being.** There are many services at the local community level that are designed to facilitate positive developments enhancing the individual and collective well-being of community residents.

For example, there are a number of educational programs in local communities whose basic objectives are self-developmental in emphasis. These may involve parenting and family life skills, health and nutrition education, personal and family financial management, job skills improvement, and self-help skills in various areas of daily living, among many others. Moreover, as we noted earlier in this chapter, many individuals engage in self-education ventures, through correspondence courses, do-it-yourself manuals, and the like.

In addition to the above examples, community service programs in the recreation and leisure area also fall within this functional category, as do community activity centers for senior citizens and young people. Furthermore, a community's library system, with its wealth of resources for personal development, ranks high as a human services mechanism of the developmental and enhancement variety.

In sum, a high proportion of a community's human services intended to respond to citizen's developmental and enhancement needs reflect the "prime community services" and "social utilities" concepts advanced by Urban and Vondracek (1977) and by Kahn (1973), respectively.

>>List some other examples of community human services of the developmental and ehancement type. What aspects of these services lead to positive and constructive individual or group development?<<

The Preventative and Institutional Modification Function

The intervention purpose of the preventative and institutional modification function of community human services is **to bring about changes in the local physical and social environment that result in improvements in the quality of life for those residing in the community.** This category, like the preceding four, is also broad in the specific types of community services it encompasses.

For example, efforts to install pollution controls that remove toxic wastes from the physical environment, health screening and "wellness" programs that combine both early health-problem identification and prevention of illness, and changes in community facilities leading to improved public sanitation are all illustrations of community human services with an underlying motive of prevention.

Local economic and industrial development programs may also fall into this category, inasmuch as many such programs are designed to prevent decline in the local economy and labor force by revitalizing techniques and attraction of new businesses into the local area.

Community service programs directed toward modifications in local institutions are often process-oriented. For example, women and other minorities may mount programs designed to change procedures resulting in discriminatory patterns in employment and wages. Other programs may employ community organizing techniques as a means of "empowering" citizen's groups as advocacy organizations to bring pressures to bear on local government officials for changes in the allocation of community services and facilities or in the processes by which community priorities are set and budgetary allocations made.

179

>>List some other community programs with preventative or institutional modification aims. Who are the intended beneficiaries of these programs? In the case of insititutional modification, who gains and who loses?<<

Conclusion

In this chapter, we have explored different dimensions of local communities and their human service systems. It should be evident at this point that, when we use the term "human services" in reference to local community contexts, we are implicitly referring to an enormous range of systems and resources to assist individuals, families, neighborhoods, and the entire community with everyday problems of human development as well as other problems of individual or group dysfunction.

Each local community is, of course, bound in many ways to larger social systems, including state and national governments, national corporate headquarters of local branch operations, and the more subtle intrusions of societal cultural values through written and visual media, as well as personal experiences through travel, both national and international.

We would contend, though, that the local commmunity, however much a part of "mass society," is still the bedrock social system in which the major part of our daily life-sustaining needs are met--some through the "prime community systems" and others through "backup community systems" which come into play when problems arise that are beyond the resources of the individual to handle.

It is also a reality that none of us deals directly with the entire human services system. As professionals in the system, or as citizens who seek to use it, we interact with those aspects of the system which are most relevant to our jobs or our needs. Furthermore, the success of any interactions with the parts will be influenced greatly by our understanding of the overall system. Thus we will examine the policymaking and decisionmaking process in the next chapter, and the nature of units and interactions in the one after that. These two chapters will provide a general framework for understanding the process and structure of community and human service systems within which specific programs and agencies operate.

Chapter IV

REFERENCES

Agranoff, Robert, ed. **Human Services on a Limited Budget.** Washington, D. C..: International City Management Association, 1983.

Agranoff, Robert, and Alex Pattakos. **Dimensions of Services Integration.** Rockville, Md.: Project SHARE, Human Services Monograph Series, No. 13, 1979.

Bates, Frederick L., and Lloyd Bacon. "The Community as a Social System," **Social Forces**, 50, March 1972, 371-379.

Bernard, Jessie. **The Sociology of Community.** Glenview, Ill.: Scott, Foresman and Company, 1973.

Borkman, Thomasina. "Experiential Knowledge: A New Concept for the Analysis of Self-Help Groups," **Social Service Review**, 50, September 1976, 445-456.

Clark, Burton. "Organizational Adaptation and Precarious Values," **American Sociological Review**, 21, 1956, 327-336.

Caplan, Gerald. **Principles of Preventive Psychiatry.** New York: Basic Books, 1964.

Collins, Alice H. "Natural Delivery Systems: Accessible Sources of Power for Mental Health," **American Journal of Orthopsychiatry**, 43, 1973, 46-52.

D'Augelli, Anthony R., Theodore R. Vallance, Steven J. Danish, Carl E. Young, and John L. Gerdes. "The Community Helpers Project: A Description of a Prevention Strategy for Rural Communities," **Journal of Prevention**, 1, Summer 1981, 209-224.

Duffee, David E. **Explaining Criminal Justice: Community Theory and Criminal Justice Reform.** Cambridge, Mass.: Oelgeschlager, Gunn & Hain, Publishers, Inc., 1980.

Durman, Eugene C. "The Role of Self-Help in Service Provision," **Journal of Applied Behavioral Science**, 12, 1976, 433-443.

Friedlander, Walter. **Introduction to Social Welfare.** Englewood Cliffs, N. J.: Prentice-Hall, Inc., 1955.

Friedson, Eliot. "Client Control and Medical Practice," **American Journal of Sociology**, 65, January 1960, 374-382.

Gates, Bruce L. **Social Program Administration.** Englewood Cliffs, N. J.: Prentice-Hall, Inc., 1980.

Gilbert, Neil, and Harry Specht, eds. **Handbook of the Social Services.** Englewood Cliffs, N. J.: Prentice-Hall, Inc., 1981.

Gottlieb, Benjamin H. "Lay Influences on the Utilization and Provision of Health Services: A Review," **Canadian Psychological Review**, 17, 1976, 126-136.

Gottlieb, Benjamin H., ed. **Social Networks and Social Support.** Beverly Hills, Calif.: Sage Publications, Inc., 1981.

Hasenfeld, Yeheskel. "People-Processing Organizations; An Exchange Approach," **American Sociological Review**, 37 June 1972, 256-263.

Hasenfeld, Yeheskel, and Richard A. English, eds. **Human Service Organizations.** Ann Arbor: The University of Michigan Press, 1974.

Hodgkinson, Virginia Ann, and Murray S. Weitzman. **Dimensions of the Independent Sector: A Statistical Profile.** Washington, D. C.: Independent Sector, 1984.

Hunter, Albert. "The Loss of Community: An Empirical Test through Replication," **American Sociological Review**, 40, October 1975, 537-552.

Huttman, Elizabeth D. **Introduction to Social Policy.** New York: McGraw Hill Publishing Co., Inc., 1981.

Jain, Sagar C., ed. **Role of State and Local Governments in Relation to Personal Health Services.** Washington, D. C.: American Public Health Association, 1981.

Jorgensen, Lou Ann B. "Social Services in Business and Industry," in **Handbook of the Social Services**, ed. Neil Gilbert and Harry Specht. Englewood Cliffs, N. J.: Prentice-Hall, Inc., 1981, pp. 337-352.

Kadushin, Charles. "The Friends and Supporters of Psychotherapy: On Social Circles in Urban Life," **American Sociological Review**, 31, December 1966, 786-801.

Kahn, Alfred J. **Social Policy and Social Services.** New York: Random House 1973.

Kammerman, Sheila B., and Alfred J. Kahn. **Social Services in the United States: Policies and Programs.** Philadelphia: Temple University Press, 1977.

Kaufman, Harold F. "Toward an Interactional Conception of Community," **Social Forces**, 38, October 1959, 9-17.

Lee, Barrett A., R. S. Oropesa, Barbara J. Metch, and Avery M. Guest. "Testing the Decline-of-Community Thesis: Neighborhood Organizations in Seattle, 1929 and 1979," **American Journal of Sociology**, 89, March 1984, 1161-1188.

Loewenberg, Frank M., and Robert Dolgoff, eds. **The Practice of Social Intervention: Goals, Roles and Strategies.** Itasca, Ill.: F. E. Peacock, Publishers, 1972.

Macarov, David. **The Design of Social Welfare.** New York: Holt, Rinehart, and Winston, 1978.

Magill, Robert S. **Community Decision Making for Social Welfare.** New York: Human Sciences Press, 1979.

Mandell, Betty Reid, and Barbara Schram. **Human Services: An Introduction.** New York: John Wiley & Sons, Inc., 1983.

March, Michael S. "The Neighborhood Center Concept," **Public Welfare**, 26, April 1968, 97-111.

Morehouse, Thomas A. **The Problem of Measuring the Impacts of Social-Action Programs.** Fairbanks: University of Alaska, Institute of Social, Economic and Government Research, 1970.

Morris, Robert. **Social Policy of the American Welfare State.** New York: Harper and Row, Publishers, 1979.

Morris, Robert. "The Human Services Function in Local Government," in **Managing Human Services**, ed. Wayne F. Anderson, Bernard J. Frieden, and Michael J. Murphy. Washington, D. C.: International City Management Association 1977, pp. 5-36.

O'Connell, Brian, ed. **America's Voluntary Spirit.** New York: The Foundation Center, 1984.

Parihar, Bageshwari. **Task-Centered Management in Human Services.** Springfield, Ill.: Charles C. Thomas, Publisher, 1984.

Perlman, Robert. **Consumers of Social Services.** New York: John Wiley and Sons, Inc., 1975.

Sauber, S. Richard. **The Human Services Delivery System.** New York: Columbia University Press, 1983.

Simon, Herbert A. **Administrative Behavior.** 3rd edition. New York: The Free Press, 1976.

Stein, Maurice R. **The Eclipse of Community: An Interpretation of American Studies.** New York: Harper and Row, Publishers, 1960.

Suttles, Gerald D. **The Social Construction of American Communities.** Chicago: University of Chicago Press, 1972.

Tourigny, Ann Ward. **Community-Based Human Service Organizations: A Conceptualization.** Unpublished doctoral dissertation, The Pennsylvania State University, 1979.

Tourigny, Ann Ward, and Joe A. Miller. "Community-Based Human Service Organizations: Theory and Practice," **Administration in Social Work,** 5, Spring 1981, 79-86.

U.S. Department of Health, Education, and Welfare. **Integration of Human Services in HEW: An Evaluation of Services Integration Projects.** Vol 1. Washington, D. C.: U. S. Department of Health, Education, and Welfare, Social and Rehabilitation Services, 1972.

U.S. Department of Health and Human Services. **Characteristics of State Plans for Aid to Families with Dependent Children.** Washington, D. C.: U. S. Department of Health and Human Services, Social Security Administration, 1981.

Urban, Hugh B., and Fred W. Vondracek, "Delivery of Human Intervention Services: Past, Present, and Future," Chapter 20 in **Life-Span Individual and Family Development,** Stella R. Goldberg and Francine Deutsch. Monterey, Calif.: Brooks/Cole Publishing Co., Inc., 1977, pp. 429-448.

Vicary, Judith R., and Henry Resnik. **Preventing Drug Abuse in the Workplace.** Rockville, Md.: National Institute on Drug Abuse, 1982.

Vinter, Robert D. "Analysis of Treatment Organizations," **Social Work,** 8, July 1965, 3-15.

Warren, Donald I. "Using Helping Networks: A Key Social Bond of Urbanites." Unpublished paper, October 1980.

Warren, Donald I. **Helping Networks: How People Cope with Problems in the Urban Community.** Notre Dame, Ind.: University of Notre Dame Press, 1981.

Warren, Roland L. **The Community in America.** 3rd ed. Chicago: Rand McNally College Publishing Company, 1978.

Warren, Roland L. "The Interorganizational Field as a Focus of Investigation," **Administrative Science Quarterly,** 12, December 1967, 396-419.

Warren, Roland L., Stephen Rose, and Anne Bergunder. **The Structure of Urban Reform.** Lexington, Mass.: Lexington Books, 1974.

Weiner, Myron E. **Human Services Management: Analysis and Applications.** Homewood, Ill.: The Dorsey Press, 1982.

Weiss, Robert S., and Martin Rein. "The Evaluation of Broad-Aim Programs: A Cautionary Case and a Moral," **The Annals,** 385, September 1969, 97-109.

COMMUNITY SYSTEMS--Hyman and Miller

Chapter V

THE ECOLOGY OF PUBLIC POLICY

AND THE POLICYMAKING SYSTEM

"States are great engines moving slowly."

—Bacon
Advancement of Learning, Bk.II.

"Government is a trust, and the officers of the government are trustees; and both the trust and the trustees are created for the benefit of the people."

—Henry Clay
Speech at Lexington, May 1829

The Source Of Policies

Community policies do not arise out of thin air. Nor are they mandated by some deity and forever set in stone. People make policies. People enforce policies. People break policies. People change policies. Community policies arise when individuals or groups seek to meet human needs or wants through community action. If all needs were fulfilled and everyone behaved properly toward others, there would be no need for policies (unless, of course, certain policies were the cause of such utopian conditions). Policies are the articulation and direction of community energies for specific human purposes. They are intended to fulfil a community need or demand; and policies have a commitment of authoritative community support to enforce implementation.

187

The Ecological Approach to Policymaking

The ecology of public policy involves **the distribution of needs, interests, and sanctions among community individuals and groups, resulting in the authoritative allocation of social values, in accordance with predominant patterns of decisionmaking and action.** From this perspective, public policy originates from needs and interests in the community environment of the policymaking system. The policymaking and implementation system, the political system, is that **aspect,** or subsystem, of overall community life that is concerned with making and enforcing **binding** policies about community goals and the allocation of group values. **Allocations of values** involve the distribution of services, resources, honors, punishments, statuses, sanctions, and opportunities.

David Easton (1965), the political scientist, postulates three levels in his general model of the political system. First, basic values related to politics and authority form a basis for the **political community.** Fundamental societal values, as explicated in Chapter II for example, are social policies which define the political community and the nature of accepted behavior. Second, the laws and procedures for making and implementing policy form a **regime.** These "rules of the game," or constitution, identify the legitimate forms of political behavior and the structure of authority--whether democratic or authoritarian, dictatorial or communal. The regime also includes specific rules on selection and replacement of leaders, who may participate in the political process and how, the legitimate process for the articulation and aggregation of needs into demands, and the acceptable forms of support and political contest. Finally, there is a set of leaders, **authorities,** who are responsible for making policies and implementing them. The authorities are the people who hold office or positions of influence--whether elected, appointed, inherited or usurped--and have the capacity to make or to be involved in making decisions which are binding on members of the community. Congress, the president and executive officers, and the courts, for example, are authorities at the federal level in the United States.

A Model of The Political System

Figure 5.1 depicts the most basic elements of Easton's model. Inputs to the system are **demands** and **support** for actions. The **decisionmaking system,** the political system, consists of the structure and interaction of authorities who make decisions and take actions in accordance with regime policies. **Outputs** are the binding **decisions and actions** about the authoritative allocation of community values.

Figure 5.1

The Political System

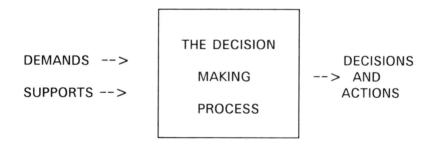

Political scientists and policy analysts have focused almost exclusively on the governmental political system. Our perspective is that this general model is useful in understanding any decisionmaking and action system. Specifically, each system has a set of fundamental values, principles or goals which are comparable to the political community—whether it be a student organization, a labor union, a family, a corporation or a governmental organization. Likewise, these systems have rules which prescribe the organizational structure, participation and decisionmaking processes—a regime. And someone is responsible for authoritative acts of the organization—whether shared and consensual among several members or manifest in a single leader. For example:

o A local probation office is guided by principles and goals which are set out in state and local statutes. The organizational structure is established by the court or department under which the office operates. The authorities are the director and his immediate superiors.

o A nonprofit community nutrition agency operates under a constitution and bylaws which set out the purposes and goals of its program. Bylaws typically also specify the rules for operation and interaction. Direction of the program would most likely come from a Board of Directors and an Executive Director.

o A motel in the hospitality industry has goals and operating principles established by its corporate charter and the purposes set out by its owner. Rules for operation include the procedures established by the owners and governmental regulations which apply. The Board of Directors and stockholders' organizations, plus top management, constitute the authorities.

o A community hospital typically has a charter which sets out its goals and purposes. It operates under procedures established by Trustees or some similar governing body, as well as rules established by appropriate government regulations. A Board of Directors and top management have the authority to make policies and decisions for the hospital.

o A neighborhood organization is typically organized for purposes specified by its members. A constitution and bylaws (formal or informal) provide for structure and interaction. An elected president and officers typically perform the roles of authorities.

>>Think about the community, regime, and authorities of a student organization in which you are involved. . . . A church. . . . Your family. . . . A university. The specific community and the content of each type of system vary, but the general model is applicable to all of these types of decisionmaking system.<<

Nadel (1975) also argues that if the policies of private organizations are "binding" on members of society, then they are authoritative (whether or not they are legitimated by governmental political authorities). Two types of bindingness which are associated with this phenomenon are **"sanction bindingness,"** and **"situation bindingness."** The former is enforced through some sort of punishment or consequence for noncompliance, or threat thereof. If you are caught speeding, the sanction may be a fine or imprisonment. If a person wants Medicare, she must comply with regulations or be denied benefits. If a person misrepresents qualifications for Medicaid, it is a punishable act. Likewise, private physicians and dentists who systematically refuse to treat medicaid recipients because the payments are too low are imposing consequences on poor people. Utility companies that shut off service in cold weather are carrying out some very binding policies which may result in hypothermia, increased risk of fires and even death. These "authorities" in both public and private sectors exercise broad powers to make and enforce sanctions beyond their specific organization and to distribute benefits. Their policies thus take on a public character.

In the case of **situation bindingness**, compliance arises from the situation of those affected--they have no direct involvement in whether the sanction will be applied to them: the options of recipients or targets of policy are controlled by the binder. You do not have the option of not paying income taxes which have already been withheld from your paycheck (Nadel, 1975) People in the Northeast and Canada cannot choose not to be affected by acid rain from industrial smokestacks. People are generally unable to control neither toxic corporate waste under their homes, nor can they choose not to consume unlabeled additives like EDB, antibotics and growth hormones which find their way into their food supply via additives in animal feed, or to avoid the effects of a "bear market" on Wall Street. Situation bindingness applies because these effects do not occur naturally or as a result of government actions; they occur as consequences of private corporate actions. Nonetheless, people in the commnity have little choice but to be bound by these policies.

Nadel illustrates his point by suggesting that the model of the policymaking process be modified from one in which the demands of community groups lead to government policy (as in Figure 5.2) to one in which policy may be made either directly or by government (as in Figure 5.3). Thus, nongovernmental organizations perform important policy and decisionmaking roles for whatever constituency they control, **and** they often function as participants in public policy in the broader societal sense.

Figure 5.2

The Governmental Policymaking Process

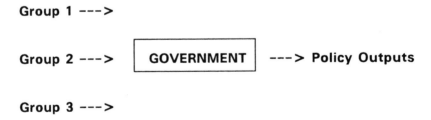

This perspective is particularly important for community and human services where it is **public policy** that many services must be provided by the voluntary and private sectors. A considerable proportion of the goods and services provided in the areas of health, social services, nutrition, family relations, services to youth and programs for the elderly are controlled not by public community standards directed to client interests, but by the standards of organizations which are concerned with profits and/or their own religious or ethical principles. This situation applies most

Figure 5.3

The Public/Private Policymaking Process

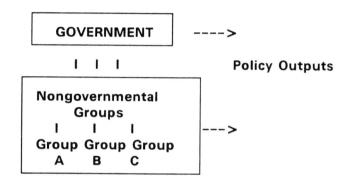

dramatically at this time when we have a national administration which is dedicated to limiting the role of government in these areas, thereby leaving people to the vicissitudes of the private/voluntary marketplace. The next sections of this chapter explicate the several aspects of community decisionmaking and action, and the elements of this general model of the policymaking system.

The Community Origin of Inputs: Demands And Support

Demands and supports originate within the community environments of the political system. People live in communities where the process of living occurs. And they frequently have needs, wants, desires, etc., which they may strive to meet through community interactions. Shared values and cultural patterns provide a basis for cohesion, cooperation and socialization (including political socialization). Differences in the attainment of values and satisfaction of needs lead to competition and conflict. Competition and conflict frequently lead like-minded· or similarly affected individuals to come together and to create groups in the community

(Dahrendorf 1959). These "interests" and "interest groups," in turn, articulate and aggregate separate wants, needs, desires, etc. (latent demands) into potential **demands** for community action--demands on the political system. They also provide reservoirs of power, influence, and resources to **support** political activity.

When the latent demands of an individual or group are communicated to authorities and gain access to the decisionmaking processes, a demand has occurred: the issue is "in" the political system for consideration. Similarly, supports include such resources as those provided by taxes, direct service as in the case of military or emergency aid, participation in campaigns to select leaders, casting votes for candidates, and less tangible supports such as patriotism and psychological support.

Several theories on related aspects of human development provide linkages between individuals and political behavior. Abraham Maslow (1954), a psychologist, theorizes that individuals have five levels of needs arranged in a "hierarchy of prepotency" as follows:

o **PHYSIOLOGICAL NEEDS,** such as hunger and thirst.

o **SAFETY NEEDS,** such as security and stability.

o **BELONGINGNESS AND LOVE NEEDS,** such as identification and affection.

o **ESTEEM NEEDS,** such as prestige and self-respect.

o **SELF-ACTUALIZATION,** or the need to develop one's potentialities in their most effective and complete form.

The more fundamental needs are necessary for **life**. And, to use a familiar phrase, we could say that the others relate to their **liberty and happiness.** Some of these needs are met by direct interaction between individuals; others are addressed by group interactions, societal organizations, or interactions with the physical environment. Growing a garden, fishing and hunting can provide food for one's immediate family, as can gainful employment. Primary group contacts (family and friends) provide for belongingness, love, etc.

Not all needs, however, are met so directly. Complex interactions in the broader community are typically necessary. Hence, social, economic, and cultural systems become involved. We can thus infer that, when people seek to have their needs met by community systems, demands for policies and actions will occur. This provides one explanation of the sources of inputs to the political system.

>>What community systems would be logical manifestations of the Maslovian needs in public policies? For example, welfare and food aid programs would meet physiological needs, while job opportunity and recreation programs would provide choices for self-actualization.<<

To test your understanding of these principles, take a few minutes to list several community subsystems and programs which might apply for each of Maslow's categories:

PHYSIOLOGICAL:

SAFETY:

BELONGINGNESS AND LOVE:

ESTEEM:

SELF-ACTUALIZATION:

The literature on needs and motivations also helps us to understand why people respond differently to different policies. A family which is living in the depths of poverty, for example, would have needs at the more basic levels--survival. To expect family members to be concerned about higher-level needs such as higher education or quality in employment may thus be inappropriate. We frequently encounter situations where people who are operating at one level of motivation do not understand, and are frustrated by, people at a different level. Furthermore, this literature helps us gain insights into one possible source of disagreement and conflict over what policies ought to be enacted and enforced. Different needs and motivations would naturally lead to different interests.

Another model which links the individual to the broader system is Talcott Parsons' "theory of action." Parsons and Shils' (1962) theory is based on the concept that individuals act in response to stimuli from the environment in the form of "artifacts" and "sociofacts." Individuals then process their perceptions of physical and social stimuli through an individual decisionmaking system wherein values, attitudes, needs, motivations, etc., provide criteria for evaluating behavior options. A choice among options leads to decisions to act or not to act. This interactional system of action suggests that some personal decisions **may** lead to community actions (inputs to the political system), while others choose do not do so.

Consider the different perceptions which might occur when a policeman, or a social worker, or an M.D., or a plumber, or you encounter an abused child along the street. What about an indigent person who walks into the church on Sunday? A banker in a blue tweed suit eating a croissant? A woman being assaulted on a pool table in a bar? A teenager acting "tipsy" in town on Saturday night? Clearly, individual perception and decisionmaking systems lead to different acts by individuals. In the highly publicized case of the barroom pool table rape, some people joined in, others stood by and watched, others cheered. Apparently no one chose to intervene or to call for help. An entire nation, however, was shocked at what occurred, and the justice system prosecuted six people, finding four guilty. Thus, individuals may act to support, deny or aggravate a need, or they may remain apathetic and distant.

>>What attitudes and values would be associated with different responses to the above situations? Do you think that people might respond differently to certain

situations, depending on which of their many value systems were brought into play? Cooperative activity and social action is frequently based on calling forth altruistic, helping and justice-related values to prompt people to act.<<

Finally, Easton (1965) specifies that inputs occur as a result of wants, needs, desires, etc., that arise as a consequence of several "environmental subsystems." The economic subsystem, the physical subsystem, the sociocultural subsystem and other governmental subsystems are sources of demands and supports for the political system. Figure 3.6 in a previous chapter depicts Easton's model of the flow of effects from community environments to the political system. The impetus for policies arises in the community, and is dependent on the interactions and decisions of individuals and groups who decide to act, or not to act, in a political manner.

>>In this framework, what would be the result of apathy or alienation? What about civil disobedience? Terrorism?<<

Note that the "systems within systems" principle applies here too. If our focal system is a specific community, then the influence of extra-community policies and groups would be extra-community inputs (and vice versa). It is useful to consider a series of ever-widening circles of system around the focal system--much like the ripples around a stone thrown into a pool of water.

The Regime And The Community

The **regime** of a policymakng system specifies the rules for decisionmaking and action. It defines the political aspect or subsystem of a community or organization. The acceptable types of demands and the process for voicing them to authorities are generally known by community members. The regime also provides means for the selection of leaders and how they are to govern. Each community or organization also has rules which delineate the accepted ways of making and implementing decisions.

>>Think about the various means for selection of leaders, e.g., voting, inheritance, corporate promotion, etc. Make your own list in the space at the left.<<

The regime also specifies the structure of authority and the distribution of power. These latter aspects of the regime influence the probability that certain demands will gain access to the decisionmaking arena and whether they will be transformed into authoritative acts. Thus the regime establishes the fundamental parameters on who gets what, when, and how.

>>What different forms of government can you name; for example, democratic, dictatorial, republic, elitist, pluralist, or communal? Plato's **Republic** presents a sixfold typology of "good" and "bad" forms of government by one, the few, and the many.<<

Conflict And The Political System

The systems perspective causes us to focus on the ways in which people come together for community action. Another perspective, represented by such conflict theorists as Ralf Dahrendorf, C. Wright Mills, Lewis Coser and Georg Simmel, addresses the role of hierarchy and power in decisionmaking and control. Conflict theorists suggest that in a situation of relative scarcity, individuals and groups seek to achieve their goals at the expense of others. The result is a hierarchical system of dominance/subordination based on power derived from economic inequities or sociocultural inequalities (class or status). We will explore these two perspectives in a later chapter.

At this point, we should say that our perspective is that these two dominant paradigms (consensus theory and conflict theory) are not incompatible, but that they address different aspects of the policymaking and enforcement phenomenon. Except for a hypothetical "war of all against all," conflict occurs within or between ongoing sociopolitical systems. Policies are necessary to guide and control human behavior whenever groups exist: they arise from the human condition of striving for survival and betterment in an imperfect world. Lack of inexhaustible resources and differences between people as to what is desirable and appropriate lead to competition and conflict. When some individuals and groups are able to achieve their goals over others and are able to acquire positions of authority to enforce them, inequities and hierarchy occur. The ecological approach to the policy process requires examination of the continuing efforts of communities to deal with past decisions which have created a given status quo, and to confront challenges for change from both the human and physical environments. As noted earlier, policies are the embodiment of the current state of the system and intended future directions, and they may emerge either as a cooperative effort by all or a result of the influence of a few.

The Authorities: Two Faces
Of The Policymaking System

The authorities are those individuals who occupy social roles which allow them to be involved in the control of inputs to and outputs from policymaking systems. Authorities play key roles in two "faces" of the political system. On the input side, authorities perform a "gatekeeping" function to decide which latent demands are allowed to enter the system. On the output side, they function as decisionmakers who make and implement policies.

Gatekeeping: The Parameters of Access

Gatekeepers decide whether **access** will occur. The wants, needs, desires, expectations . . . of citizens do not automatically become demands, nor do they enter the system in some mysterious or mystical way. Demands are created only as members of the political community articulate wants in a way which indicates that they feel the wants ought to be handled by binding policies (Easton, 1965, p. 81). Access requires that supporters of latent demands seek to approach or gain admission to the policymaking process to satisfy the demands, **and** that such wants come to the "attentive interest of the relevant decisionmakers."

> . . . [The] concept of access must be clearly distinguished from the concept of power. Access should be regarded as the measurable (in principle) probability that if the members of a group or its leaders perceive an interest affected by a future authoritative decision, the group can obtain the **attentive interest** of the relevant decisionmakers. Access thus describes a continuum of behavior situations: at the one end, the group has no access, (and no power) regardless of whether it perceives an interest or not; in the middle, if the group perceives an interest, it can act--it has effective access; at the other end--the maximum preferred goal of all interest groups--the group has privileged access. Privileged access can be defined as the probability that authoritative decisionmakers automatically take a group's interests into account. (Scoble 1968)

Gatekeeping, the capacity to grant access, does not automatically lead to decisions or actions. Each political system or organization has norms and rules which define who gets different degrees of access, the type of demands which get in, and the probability of successful conversion to policies.

In small communities, face-to-face groups, committees and simple societies where social and political roles are not highly differentiated, almost everyone can act as a gatekeeper: membership qualifies one to raise issues, and to have them considered. Where a high degree of structural division of labor prevails, gatekeeping tends to go to the incumbents of specialized roles. Elites, well-organized interest groups, community influentials, and political leaders tend to carry out the gatekeeping role. Thus, in different situations, all of the following tend to provide means to access: (1) the selection of elites and leaders, (2) membership in elites, (3) interest group pressures, (4) direct mass pressure, (5) indirect pressure through the media and public opinion, and (6) individual pleas to incumbents of authority roles. Thus, in simple systems, access too is relatively easy; in more complex systems, access takes on more differentiated and complex characteristics.

>>Who are the gatekeepers in your family? Are there certain topics that your parents won't even discuss (nondecisions)?

Who is the gatekeeper of a college class? What are the rules for raising demands about changing course schedules, examinations, or term paper topics?

How would one go about getting an item on the agenda of the student government? How about the city council? List the gatekeepers in each situation in the space at the left.<<

The Other Face: Decisionmakers

Decisionmakers are those individuals whose roles include responsibility for the **outputs** of the political system. The three output functions of any political system are: **rule-making, rule-application, and rule-adjudication.** These functions were articulated by Almond and Coleman (1960) to generalize what are usually referred to as the legislative, executive and judicial "branches of government."

Rule-making involves the establishment or revision of binding policies, procedures, laws or rules. Legislatures, city councils, and corporate and organization boards of directors generally carry out this function at the highest level of an organization. Agency staff and others, however, are involved in making more specific rules about regulations and procedures. Thus all "branches," and all levels of the policymaking system have some involvement in rule-making.

>>What authority would make the following rules:

-Police officers in St. Louis are required to take an annual competency examination.

-Nurses in Mercy Hospital may administer prescription drugs on their own professional judgment.

-Adults without dependent-age children may receive only three months of financial assistance from the state's public welfare system in any annual period.

-Instructors must inform each of their university classes of the rules governing academic honesty and integrity.

-People receiving utility service must pay or be cut off--even in the dead of winter.

-A neighborhood community services agency provides shelter

assistance for one night only to needy individuals.

—Fraternity XKN has a two-beer limit for parties.

—Joe Albertson will not loan his car on either football or party weekends.<<

Rule-application refers to the application of rules to specific situations. The delivery of services, social protection, and the assurance of rights and entitlements are applications of policies. The rule-application function is typically carried out by the executive agencies of a government, or by the administrative staff of a private corporation or voluntary organization. Rule-application is the implementation of policies.

>>Who would be responsible for application of the rules identified above?<<

Rule-adjudication occurs when disputes arise between actors in the political process. For example, individuals may disagree with service delivery personnel over decisions about eligibility or benefits. Groups and corporations may disagree about the application or interpretation of laws or regulations. The courts are primary arbiters of conflicts; however, administrative hearings and various forms of mediation, arbitration and advocacy provide for the involvement of other agencies as well.

>>Who would adjudicate the following disputes?

—Mrs. Crookedneck requests $100,000 damages from Mr. Driver for alleged pain and suffering from an auto accident. Mr. Driver denies responsibility and declines to pay.

203

-Mr. Fury asks for custody of the children, contending that his wife is an abusive and unfit parent.

-Mr. Picayune contends that his conviction for armed robbery was a frame-up and that the evidence was concocted by the police.

-Miss Etudiante disputes her landlord's eviction notice which is based on an allegation of loud parties and damage to the apartment.

-Mr. Bell contends that he should not have to pay for the long distance charges on his telephone bill because they were made by his roommate.

-Mrs. Mendicant believes that she has been wrongfully denied food stamps.

-Miss Stone disagrees with the medication being given her by the hospital physician.<<

Opposition Within The Authorities

In democratic systems the hierarchy of authority is such that the ruling elite, or "authorities," include members who have varying degrees of agreement with those who are incumbents of the dominant positions. Different parties or factions continually vie for dominance. There are degrees of cooperation and conflict within the ruling group, e.g., Democrats, Republicans, Independents and others in U.S. politics. In campus government there may be dormies, townies, frats, jocks, eggheads and minority groups. In human service systems there are divisions within and disagreements between different professions, as well as across different subsystems.

The political process provides a nonviolent arena for resolving disputes and conflicts over which demands are to be met, and to what degree. The outcome of these conflicts determines whether policies will be made and implemented to resolve the demands (wants, needs, desires, etc.) of community groups, and when specific supports (taxes or service) will be required. In a situation of scarce resources, choices will be made which lead to some being benefited and others being denied. The structure of power, authority and influence; the overall social values and subsystem policies; and the regime policy of the current administration are dominant influences on the outcomes. The impact of changes will be reflected in new conditions, met or unmet expectations, or changes of the broader community, which in turn determine whether new or continuing latent demands exist--and the cycle continues.

The Relationship To Systems in General

It is important at this point to recall the principles of general systems mentioned in an earlier chapter. Specifically, the "systems within systems" principle allows us to consider different levels of a larger system as subsystems. In turn, each subsystem may be considered a system in its own right. As applied here, we can understand that the different sectors of community systems and various human service programs all perform the functions of a political system--but each in its specific domain. It is relatively easy to understand how a government provides these functions, for we have been socialized to this perspective. Consider a specific human service agency with which you are familiar--how do the various concepts apply? Service "intake and eligibility" personnel perform the "access" function. Disputes may be handled by supervisors or a separate "fair hearing" process in the organization. Interpretations of directives from higher levels are a form of rule-making, as are the detailed local guidelines and procedures. Thus, the model of the political process explicated in this chapter will prove useful as we consider the structure and units of human services in American communities in the next chapter.

Chapter V

REFERENCES

Almond, Gabriel, and James S. Coleman. **The Politics of the Developing Areas.** Princeton, N. J.: Princeton University Press, 1960.

Dahl, Robert A. **Who Governs?** New Haven: Yale University Press, 1961.

Dahrendorf, Ralf. **Class and Class Conflict in Industrial Society.** Stanford, Calif.: Stanford University Press, 1959.

Easton, David. **A Systems Analysis of Political Life.** N. Y.: John Wiley and Sons, 1965.

Maslow, Abraham H. **Motivation and Personality.** N. Y.: Harper, 1954.

Mills, C. Wright. **The Power Elite.** N. Y.: Oxford University Press, 1956.

Nadel, Mark. "The Hidden Dimension of Public Policy: Private Governments and the Policy-Making Process." **The Journal of Politics,** Vol. 37, 1975, pp. 1-34.

Ostrom, Vincent. **Polycentricity.** American Political Science Association, 1972 Annual Meeting, paper.

Parsons, Talcott, and Edward Shils. **Toward a General Theory of Action.** N. Y.: Harper and Row, 1962.

Parsons, Talcott. **Systems and Process in Modern Societies.** N. Y.: The Free Press, 1960.

Polyani, Michael. **The Logic of Liberty.** Chicago: University of Chicago Press, 1951.

Scoble, Harry M. "Access to Politics." **International Encyclopedia of the Social Sciences.** Vol. 1. N. Y.: MacMillan Co., 1960, pp. 10-14.

Chapter VI

OUR POLYCENTRIC SYSTEM:
SIMULTANEOUS GAMES AND MULTIPLE ARENAS

"A truly chaotic state of affairs would not persist over time
unless a Grand Randomizer were available to "maintain" a
chaotic "order."

-Ostrom
Polycentricity

"The appearance of disorder which prevails on the surface
leads one at first to imagine that society is in a state of
anarchy nor does one perceive one's mistake till one has gone
deeper into the subject."

-Alexis de Toqueville
Democracy in America

The Structure of Authority

The conventional model of the political system depicts a
continuous process of decisionmaking from the generation of latent
demands by actors in the community, through input of demands to
the authorities, to conversion of the demands into authoritative
decisions and allocations of values for the community. The products
or outputs of this system are policies which guide and direct the
decisions and actions of authorities in rule-making, rule-application
and rule-adjudication. This general model of the political system
provides a framework for understanding the elements and process of
policymaking and implementation. The model seems to imply,
however, that policies are made and carried out by a system with a
rational structure of authority organized hierarchically.

209

It is generally agreed, however, that in the United States authority and the capacity to make and enforce binding policies are highly diffused into multiple jurisdictions. These different spheres of authority are frequently competing and overlapping, and highly dynamic in their interactions. The structures for the allocation of community values have evolved over several hundred years in response to various historical crises, issues and events. The result is a highly complex pattern of sociopolitical structures in the community whereby policies and authority, as discussed in earlier chapters, are divided along several dimensions: (1) **community value subsystem,** including health, employment, housing, transportation, education, and similar areas of local concern; (2) **level of jurisdiction** (or locality), including township, city, county, state, borough, regional, national, neighborhood, association, or corporation; and (3) **sector,** including the public, voluntary, and private sectors. The result is a policy system which is characterized by thousands of separate, competing jurisdictions which divide, shift and coalesce according to the exigencies of the moment. (For example, there are over 2,000 separate police departments and over 500 school districts in the State of Pennsylvania alone.)

This chapter examines several key dimensions of the structure of authority of community systems in America. The types of **actors** or **units** in community systems are delineated, and the several **sectors** of organization are defined. These concepts form the bases for a typology of community actors which provides a framework for analyzing, planning, organizing and managing community and human service systems.

Polycentricity vs. Monocentricity

Michael Polyani (1951) and Vincent Ostrom (1972) characterize the American system of authority as "polycentric." A **polycentric** system is depicted as one in which many actors, each possessing a degree of decisional autonomy (i.e., authority over some or all aspects of a jurisdiction), "participate in a series of simultaneous games and where each act has the potential for being a move in simultaneous games." (Ostrom, 1972, p. 5) The polycentric system is contrasted to a **monocentric** system, which has a single center of authority and direction. Centralized polities, bureaucracies and most corporations are organized hierarchically with authority flowing from a single source. Many "focal systems" or programs in community systems also have monocentric structures. The overall system in American communities, however, does not generally reflect the monocentric form; thus, it is to the polycentric form that this chapter is directed.

The process of decisionmaking and action in a polycentric system is characterized by continual shifts in the roles and relationships among actors. Consider, for example, the provision of services to the poor and disadvantaged in Pennsyulvania, a state in which the Public Welfare has the responsibility for many human service programs, but in most cases, shares authority and responsibility with other jurisdictions.

Cash assistance, or cash supplements for families with dependent children and employable single adults is provided through sixty-seven county boards of assistance (CBAs) which are administered by the state Department of Public Welfare, drawing on state funds and supported from federal grants through the Social Security Act. Similar aid for disabled and elderly people, however, is provided directly to individuals by federal social security programs. There are also federal food stamps and surplus food which are provided through a federal Department of Agriculture Program, with the former administered by the CBAs and the latter by local voluntary service agencies. In addition, there are thousands of private charities and religious organizations which provide cash and/or in-kind aid. Certain types of education grants and loans also provide financial assistance for students through a state higher education assistance agency and private banks.

Employment and vocational rehabilitation services are required for people on cash assistance, but these services are provided through two separate bureaus of the Department of Labor and Industry. The Welfare department, however, administers a Commonwealth

Neighborhood Careers Program, which provides jobs in state institutions, and a Youth Corps Program for young people. Additionally, there are many private employment services as well as direct contacts by job seekers with employers which allocate this value. Furthermore, most social service agencies also regard employment services as part of their mandate.

Social services are the responsibility not only of the sixty-seven separate, state-administered CBA's, but also of the sixty-seven separate county-administered children and youth agencies (which are only "supervised" by the State Department of Public Welfare). There are also sixty-seven juvenile probation offices administered by the county courts to deal with juvenile delinquency cases. Moreover, there are thousands of social service agencies in the "voluntary sector" under the aegis of private charities, religious organizations, Health and Welfare Councils, United Funds, and professional associations. These latter organizations may or may not fall under state regulations or guidelines, and may or may not receive public funds.

In the area of **housing and living conditions,** the private marketplace provides the main structures for allocation, although there are various agencies regulating building and real estate transactions, and there are various levels of public health, zoning and building inspections. Public housing is typically provided by local housing authorities, although funding and regulations come through federal FHA, VA, Community Development Block Grants and the Housing Assistance Act. In addition, housing assistance for the aged, blind and disabled is a shared responsibility among the private market, county, state and voluntary sectors, although the Department of Public Welfare has general licensing responsibilities. County homes are also provided for the aged indigent, and foster care and group homes are available for children through county and private child welfare programs. Temporary private shelter is frequently provided by churches and social agencies.

Mental health and mental retardation services are provided both through thousands of private medical entrepreneurs for whom the state has licensing responsibility. The state also operates institutions for the mentally ill and state schools for the retarded through the Department of Public Welfare. Forty-two Community Mental Health–Mental Retardation Programs (single county or multi-county "joinders") are administered by the sixty-seven counties, subject to the regulations and the annual approval of a plan by the State Department of Public Welfare and federal regulations. Many county (or multi-county) MH/MR Programs receive direct federal aid, as well as local funding.

Medical services are generally available in the marketplace. Payments for medical services for low-income citizens are available through State Department of Public Welfare under its version of medical assistance, and supported by federal medical assistance (Medicaid). Elderly people are similarly covered in part by the federal Medicare Program. County nurses and regional well-baby clinics are State Department of Health programs. The welfare department operates several state-owned general hospitals, however, and also administers the federal Hill-Burton hospital construction program. (Hyman, 1975)

While extremely complex, this example actually presents a simplified account of the organization and funding for **some** of the human services available to people in Pennsylvania. This rather extended illustration serves not only to depict the multiplicity of juridictions which obtain in a single state but also to point out that it is **public policy** that these conditions exist. **In such a system, every unit or member has authority over some aspects of individual/community life, although the ramifications for other systems and the total system will vary greatly.** Talcott Parsons comments on this phenomenon:

In these terms every subsystem within the society has its patterns of authority because on its own level every subsystem has political functions and differential political responsibility. But these will differ for different types of subsystems within the society, by the various criteria by which authority patterns can and do vary. (Parsons 1960)

Many observers of the American system interpret the existence of fragmentation of authority and overlapping jurisdictions as irrational, chaotic, and not amenable to systematic understanding. It is our observation, however, that individuals and organizations continue to operate, to survive, and even to prosper under these conditions. Most importantly, they understand how to do so, and polycentric systems are usually negotiated with considerable efficiency. In response to observations about the "irrationality" of the system, Ostrom states the following:

Presumably a truly chaotic state of affairs would not persist over time unless a Grand Randomizer were available to "maintain" a chaotic "order." Furthermore, a truly chaotic state can hardly be evaluated by performance criteria such as efficiency or responsiveness. For a polycentric political system to exist and persist through time, a structure of ordered relationships would have to prevail, perhaps, under an illusion of chaos. If such a structure of ordered relationships exists, one might assume that specifiable structural conditions will evoke predictable patterns of conduct. (Ostrom, 1972, p. 5)

To begin understanding the polycentric system within which community human service systems operate, we shall need to understand the actors or units of action, the sectors of action, and the interunit/interorganizational relationships which exist. The next sections of this chapter address these topics.

Actors And
Units Of Action

The community systems perspective recognizes that units of action may be individuals, groups, or organizations. This orientation is based on the concept that integrated systems or patterns of behavior of groups of individuals or organizations have qualities which make them more than simply the sum of the individuals that are members. Such units can neither be derived from the individual units or components of which they are comprised, nor are they simply the sum of the parts. This **gestalt** perspective allows us to view a system as more than the sum of its parts. We thus define five types of units, or actors, in community systems:

>**INDIVIDUALS** acting in specific roles.

>**QUASI-GROUPS** as latent, potential or emergent groups. Not a group or entity in the sociological sense, quasi-groups are comprised of individuals who share some characteristic or interest in common which may lead them to form definite groups. They are important for our consideration because decisionmakers frequently antici-pate
the action of such "latent" interests.

>**PRIMARY GROUPS** of individuals acting in concert according to some value or goal. Groups, in the sociological sense, involve numbers of people in regular communication and with a regular structure. The interests in quasi-groups are made "manifest."

>**FORMAL ORGANIZATIONS** are secondary groups which are organized, hierarchically structured, and directed to a particular mission, goal or function.

>**WHOLE SYSTEMS** encompass general controlling or policymaking bodies of a community or subsystem such as federal and state governments, county and municipal general governments, intercorporate and multinational

215

corporations. (This is generally the "focal system" for analysis discussed earlier.)

>**THE TOTAL SYSTEM** includes not only an organization or subsystem, but also the environmental systems which impinge upon it, and the interorganizational field.*

Note that these five types of units tend to be differentiated by size and degree of formalization, as well as by scope of control. Note also, however, that the categories do not necessarily form a continuum from individual to community to state and national levels. This distinction is both purposeful and important, for the reality of community systems is based on one's location of action or analysis; this is an application of the "systems-within-systems" principle.

> >How does the following aphorism apply here? "Where you stand depends upon where you sit."< <

For illustrative purposes, let us think about a college class as a system. It is comprised of individuals acting in the roles of students and professor(s). There are most likely other resources such as a room, chairs and desks, etc. When the individuals are in the room, does the class exist? Not necessarily! The same individuals in that room could be a conspiracy, a party, a helping organization, or any number of other "units" in the broader community. Or, they might simply be a bunch of separate people in the room, each doing her or his own thing. It is not only the individual units, but the fact that they **interact** in certain ways, according to certain **rules** of interaction, and with some generally understood **purpose** that makes a **system** exist.

The class most likely has many different types of people: "brains," average students, and "nerds," for example. There may be some "jocks," "frats," "townies," and "vets." And there may be blacks,

----

* This categorization draws upon several sources: Dahrendorf (1959), Parsons (1960), Cox et al., (1974), and van Gigch (1974).

216

WASP's, Puerto Ricans, international students and other racial and ethnic groups. Generally these characteristics are not manifest in classroom dynamics--the interests based on these characteristics are **latent**. These are **quasi-groups**.

If, however, some event arises which leads people from a quasi-group to join together on a class-related issue, an **interest group** may form. For example, if a major test is scheduled for the Monday after a big "Spring Week" celebration, the "frats" may organize to ask for a change in test date; or, international students may find themselves at a disadvantage if the professor assumes considerable familiarity with the American system and may join together to try to deal with the issue.

The class itself is a **formal organization**. Students and faculty are hierarchically structured according to certain rules of interaction. An "authority" exists. And there is a purpose--even though perhaps ill-defined--of gaining/imparting knowledge about a particular topic. The class is also most likely a part of larger formal organizations--the department, college and university. Moreover, the University is part of a larger, **whole system**. A state university, for example, is part of the education system of a state. It exists and operates in the broader, whole system context of state politics. Finally, all exist within a **total system,** with other whole systems and subsystems as environmental actors.

>>Consider the various types of systems involved in the situations presented in Chapter 1. Then, try to identify the systems that are involved in producing a fast-food taco? How about a foster care home? A heart transplant? A drunk driving arrest?<<

As you become more familiar with applying systems principles, you will be able to work with these concepts at different levels of application. Thus, any subsystem might be considered in several contexts: as a focal system, as a subsystem of a broader system, or as part of the environment of another focal system. The difference depends on the focus of orientation or analysis. In the example above, a classroom was the focal unit. We might well have started with a college within the university or the university itself. In such cases, the specific content of the levels will change. This fact has led some of us to describe the system as "kaleidoscopic"--it looks different depending on your perspective, similar to the way the elements of a kaleidoscope present a different visage as the colored chips reflect light from different directions.

Figure 6.1 presents a "matrix" of community interactions based on the six types of community units. That is, it shows all of the possible types of interactions between the various types of actors, or units, in community systems. For example, an individual requesting service from a hospital involves an "individual to formal organization" interaction. An arrest of a citizen by a police officer is an interaction by a formal organization (the police department) to an individual. (Note that for purposes of this chart we have combined the "whole system" and "total system" categories into the "larger aggregates" category.) Some of the most frequent interactions in community systems and human services are:

Individual and/or primary group to:

> **Other individuals and/or primary groups.** These face-to-face interactions comprise the "lay helping network(s)" of communities and neighborhoods.

> **Formal organizations.** Individuals, families or small groups place demands on formal organizations for services or changes in programs.

> **Larger Aggregates.** Direct contact with authorities or interest groups at the total or whole system level; for example, mayors, congressmen, chief executives; corporate leadership (especially extra-community actors on the vertical dimension of power and control.)

Figure 6.1

Matrix of Community Units and Interactions

INTERACTION FROM:	INTERACTION TO:				
	INDIVIDUALS (Roles)	QUASI-GROUPS	PRIMARY GROUPS	FORMAL ORGANIZATIONS	LARGER AGGREGATES
INDIVIDUALS (Roles)				Requests for Service	Individual Appeal to Legislator or Governor's Office
QUASI-GROUPS					
PRIMARY GROUPS			Group to Group	Group to Organization Family to Social Service Agency	
FORMAL ORGANIZATIONS	Direct Service Delivery		Community Development Department Self-Help Group to Community	Neighborhood Organization to City Planning Department	Department of Welfare to Legislature
LARGER AGGREGATES		Legislature Establishes Anti-Discrimination Policy	Governor Meets with Representatives of Groups	Congress Investigates and Receives Testimony on a Social Problem	State Governor's Office to Congressional Committee

Formal organizations to:

Individuals and/or primary groups. Agencies, programs, or interest groups reach out to provide services or in other ways affect or place restrictions on individuals and primary groups.

Other formal organizations. Interorganizational relations--agencies interacting to try to change, coordinate, support, review or oppose the actions of other organizations.

Larger Aggregates. Contact between community agencies and higher authorities (total or whole system levels) for funding, appeals of regulations, demands for regulations or approval to act in specified ways.

From larger aggregate to:

Individuals and/or primary groups: Direct action from the total or whole system level to the grassroots level to circumvent intervening levels of the system; for example, direct grants to individuals.

Formal organizations. Usually directions, control, regulation, evaluation and/or funding from total or whole system levels to community agencies.

Larger aggregates. Total- or whole-system level interorganizational relations involving conflict or cooperation over policy, laws, jurisdiction, funding, etc.

Examples of some of these types of interactions are noted on the chart in Figure 6.1. After you have perused the chart, locate where each of the following would be placed:

o   A father hugs his child today.

o   A child snatches a lady's purse.

o   A policeman, acting in an official capacity, arrests the child.

o   Two low-income families get together to share resources.

o   A local housing authority takes action to protect a minority group, even though the latter is not organized as an interest group.

o   A local community mental health center applies for a direct federal grant.

o   A local community mental health center applies to the local United Way for a grant.

o   A national fast food corporation develops a marketing program to appeal to teenagers.

o   A community nutrition program presents a workshop for local families

o   A local family applies to a national restaurant chain for a franchise.

o   A county visiting nurse program provides hospice services to Mr. Jones.

o   Union County and Centre County create a "joinder" to provide child neglect and abuse services.

Specification of these different types of actors and the many types of interaction that may occur allows us to define the **units** of interaction for community systems, and to understand that a great deal of the **interaction** which occurs involves entities other than

221

individuals. Individuals acting in **roles** are, in effect, the spokespersons or communicating units of groups or formal organizations. In this way, we can refer to programs, organizations, groups, and the like as **units** of action in community systems, thus greatly simplifying our analysis.

Sectors Of Organization

Another important dimension of system units in the American federal system is the **sector** of action. Earlier, Chapters I-IV (above) introduced this concept as integral to communities and human service systems in the United States. We commonly refer to the public, voluntary and private sectors as follows:

>**PRIVATE SECTOR,** or proprietary, organizations are those which offer services in the open market for a fee. A goal of these organizations is to make a profit by providing a service which individuals and groups in communities are willing and able to pay for directly.

>**VOLUNTARY SECTOR,** or not-for-profit, agencies operate on a nonprofit basis. Staff may receive salaries for work performed, but the agency does not seek financial gain. Charitable organizations such as the United Way, Voluntary Action Centers, and a variety of clinics and social service agencies are organized to provide services to individuals and groups in the community. Services are typically free to those unable to pay, and a sliding scale may be used where some payment is possible. (This "sector" is sometimes included as part of the "private" sector.)

> **PUBLIC SECTOR,** or governmental, agencies are those operated by one or more levels of government. Public funds, generated through taxes, support these agencies. Authority to operate is derived from statutes, laws or regulations which are enforceable by public authorities.

Despite the appearance of clear distinctions between the three "sectors" and the agencies which comprise them, considerable fuzziness and blurring exist. Nadel (1975) cites four aspects to the "tenuous and artificial" distinctions. First, extensive cooperation exists between the sectors. The "public" health care programs of Medicare and Medicaid are simply payment programs for services delivered through private, voluntary **and** public providers. Government grants to private and voluntary agencies underwrite a considerable proportion of the social service, mental health, and housing programs for low-income citizens. Contracts between government and organizations in the other sectors provide much of the research, development, planning and evaluation which occur in American communities.

Second, actions of private and voluntary agencies frequently have a public policy outcome. Voluntary agencies that use a governmental "poverty line" as their own eligibility criterion are one example. Private corporations may affect public policies through plant closings, pollution, and safety practices and through the exercise of influence over local organizations.

Third, government delegates considerable power to private and voluntary organizations. Most human services professionals are policed by member associations. The American Medical Association, the National Association of Social Workers, the American Psychological Association and a plethora of others establish and may enforce most standards. These groups dominate the professional licensing functions of government, provide the standards for examinations, and stand guard over the rules for admission to and practice of the professions.

Fourth, the influence of private elites over all aspects of life, both public and private, further complicates the picture. While a controversial aspect of the private/public nexus, elitist theory contends that a "ruling class" wields effective power over public policy. Whether a "military-industrial complex" as articulated by President Dwight Eisenhower in his farewell address, or a "strategic elite" of top leaders and interlocking corporation directorates, the existence of such a dynamic would indicate considerable private influence over public policy. Furthermore, in many communities a dominant corporation or family may effectively wield enough influence to dictate public policy and affect the operation of many public organizations.

Organizational charters and tax statements may project a picture of a strict distinction between the sectors. The reality of the system, however, may reflect more of a continuum with varying degrees of public/private involvement in any one function or service. It will be useful, however, to maintain the distinctions used in the field as we continue the discussion of types of units.

A Typology Of Actors

By combining the concepts of units and sectors as presented in the preceeding two sections, we can derive a typology of actors in community human service systems (Figure 6.2).

This typology enables us to sort out key aspects of the source of authority and jurisdiction of key actors in community systems, and to define the structure of the various human service subsystems. For example, a community mental health system may have state regulation and support (public) for a county-based "base service unit" (BSU), which may be either public or private according to previous county government plans and state approvals. The actual delivery of services, though, may occur directly through the BSU or through arrangements via compacts, contracts or grants to other public, voluntary or private organizations. Furthermore, mental health services may be completely independent of the BSU, provided by voluntary or private organizations in the marketplace; or they may be operated by some other governmental unit. In Pennsylvania, for example, public state mental hospitals provide inpatient care separate from, though frequently used by, the community mental health programs. Place the following examples in the appropriate spaces in Figure 6.2.

- o **A physician in private practice.**
- o **A volunteer worker for the Red Cross.**
- o **A local housing inspector (city employee).**
- o **Consumers who use Tylenol.**
- o **A state Welfare Department worker.**
- o **Nonorganized public school teachers.**

Figure 6.2

A Typology of Community Actors

	PRIVATE SECTOR	VOLUNTARY SECTOR	PUBLIC SECTOR
INDIVIDUALS			
QUASI-GROUPS			
PRIMARY GROUPS			
FORMAL ORGANIZATIONS			
WHOLE SYSTEM (FOCAL SYSTEM)			
TOTAL SYSTEM			

o **A nuclear family.**
o **A city probation officer.**
o **United States Steel Corporation.**
o **The Salvation Army.**
o **The Department of Health**.

The "systems within systems" concepts can be used in applying this classification scheme to different "levels" of the system; for example, family, neighborhood, local community, state, region, and so forth. The concept of **focal system,** introduced earlier provides a starting point for analysis and a way of systematically organizing inquiry into the nature of a particular program or agency and its place in the broader system(s). The idea of **polycentricity** enables us to understand that many centers of authority and jurisdiction may exist and be relevant to a specific focal organization. Keep in mind also that each of the different subsystems and sub-subsystems will have both horizontal ties to other units and vertical ties to one or several other subsystems.

Social control, for example, is generally maintained by family, group, and individual-to-individual interactions in communities. The major formal organizations of social control at the local level are the various police agencies which are authorized at city, borough, or township levels (although federal and state levels provide for constitutional and statutory restrictions and extra-local guidance and directions to prevent unfettered application of force). The authority structure of such local units typically has few horizontal or vertical dimensions outside of the local jurisdiction except where multiunit agreements or metropolitan organizations are created by the relevant political units. Extra-local social control and police services typically occur through county sheriffs, state police, the FBI, the U.S. Treasury Department and similar organizations. Each of these latter organizations has its designated sphere of authority which is generally intended to deal with a separate area of policy. However, gaps may occur, leaving areas outside of control, and overlaps create duplications requiring coordination and/or generate competition and conflict. Thus, the **whole system** of a **local focal police organization** includes a variety of horizontal and vertical relationships; and the **total system** includes the full range of community subsystems--educational, income maintenance, social

226

services, cultural and recreational, etc. The system models presented in Chapters III and V provide useful guides to analysis of any system if the "authorities" are considered to be those of a focal organization.

Thus far, we have introduced the concepts of policy, system and community. Human service systems have been defined and delineated, and the systems of policymaking and control have been explained. This chapter focused on the organization of the overall system and the character of specific units. In the next chapters we turn to a consideration of basic paradigms of Western thought and their relationship to policymaking, planning, organizing-implementing and managing community systems. The themes of consensus and conflict flow throughout these subsequent chapters.

Chapter VI

REFERENCES

Cox, Fred M., John L. Ehrlich, Jack Rothman and John E. Tropman, eds. **Strategies of Community Organization.** Itasca, Ill.: F. E. Peacock Publishers, Inc., 1974

Dahrendorf, Ralf. **Class and Class Conflict in Industrial Society.** Stanford, Calif.: Stanford University Press, 1959, esp. Chapter V.

Hyman, Drew. **Citizen's Advocacy and Political Responsiveness in a Polycentric Political System.** Los Angeles, Calif: University of California, 1975.

Nadel, Mark. "The Hidden Dimension of Public Policy: Private Governments and the Policy-Making Process." **The Journal of Politics,** 37, 1975, 1-34.

Ostrom, Vincent. **Polycentricity.** American Political Science Association, 1972 Annual Meeting, paper.

Parsons, Talcott. **Systems and Process in Modern Societies.** N. Y.: The Free Press, 1960.

Polyani, Michael. **The Logic of Liberty.** Chicago, Ill.: University of Chicago Press 1951.

van Gigch, John. **Applied General Systems Theory.** N. Y.: Harper and Row, 1974.

CHAPTER VII

PLANNING AND MANAGING COMMUNITY SYSTEMS I: CONSENSUS, CONFLICT AND THE PROGRAMMING MODEL

"I love it when a plan comes together."
—Col. Hannibal Smith
The "A Team"

Proactive Change in the Polycentric System

Can one rationally plan and manage community systems in our "kaleidoscopic," polycentric system? Or is this "vast non-system" which has grown up like Topsy so diverse and dynamic that one must simply "go with the flow"? The answer to each of these qustions is "Yes, . . . depending on your perspective." The "A-Team" show can be seen as a parody of planning. Col. Smith always gives the impression that he has a plan, and that final outcomes result from the plan. In between, there is an apparently chaotic series of unforeseeable actions by the "bad guys," and irrational behavior by all of the characters involved. The planning which occurs, and the mangement of that plan, must deal not only with rationally prospective behavior, but also with a great deal of "irrationality" both within the organization and from the environment.

229

Planning and management of community services has elements of this interposition of idea and reality. This chapter looks at the issues of planning, implementation and management from two perspectives. The counterposition of the consensus perspective and the conflict perspective provides an overall theme which pervades our discussion.

Consensus and Conflict: Two Dominant Paradigms

Two dominant paradigms, or approaches, to looking at the world which have evolved in Western thought provide a basis for examining major issues in the field. Each has a characteristic way of observing and analyzing the world. Each perspective leads to different theories about the fundamental premises of how systems operate, and what makes some systems persist and others change. And each has its own recipe for how to plan, to implement programs, and to manage them. A basic understanding of these two approaches will enable you to begin to sort out the diversity and controversy which exists in the field, and to develop your own understanding of why some systems work as planned and develop effective programs, while others do not. Our objective is to enable your interactions in community systems to be not merely reactive behavior in response to other actors and environmental events, but to be **proactive,** directed to meaningful outcomes.

The Concept of Ideal Types

As indicated above, the consensus and conflict perspectives have deep roots in human thought. In Western philosophy and science, fundamental differences between Plato and Aristotle, Rousseau and Hobbes, and Weber and Marx can be seen to revolve around the question of whether human societies are rooted in rationality, consensus and shared values, or whether they are characterized by caprice, constraint and conflict. While some Eastern philosophies embrace the contraposition of opposites in the "Yin-Yang"--that is, good vs. evil, right vs. wrong, consensus vs.

conflict--Western thought has tended to drift in one direction or the other. Thus, our discussion will begin by identifying the different approaches as "ideal types," which will aid us in distinguishing the differences, and in understanding the simultaneous existence of both.

The concept of **"ideal types"** was articulated by Max Weber (1947) to distinguish dominant modes of understanding. He suggested that meaning may be derived from both **idea and experience.** One mode is based on rationally derived thoretical principles, and the other is rooted in the experiences, observations and feelings of individuals.

> The basis for certainty in understanding can be either rational, which can be further subdivided into logical and mathematical, or it can be of an emotionally empathic or artistically appreciative quality. In the sphere of action things are rationally evident chiefly when we attain a completely clear intellectual grasp of the action-elements in their intended context of meaning. (Weber, 1947, pp. 90-91)

An ideal type, then, is a theoretically generalized statement about the principles of an idea or object. It is easier to teach a youngster about the primary colors of red, blue and yellow by pointing out brightly colored flowers, clothing, stoplights, etc., to develop an understanding of the concept of "color." Then distinctions such as aquamarine, mauve, heliotrope, beige and magenta may be made; and "color" can be conceptually distinguished from other qualities of objects. Likewise, we recognize that reality is an incredibly complex web of subsystems and interactions. In order to facilitate understanding that web, particularly its constituent parts, we separate our observations into analytic categories. By focusing on the polar opposite ideal types of consensus theory and conflict theory, we will both identify their fundamental characteristics and gain an understanding of their meaning when applied to the arena of action.

Weber, in fact, recognized the action potential of ideal types. While pure theories may be constructed to facilitate understanding, they may also become **normative guides** to actions and evaluation. Individuals, organizations and groups may base their actions upon, and judge the behavior of others by comparison to, ideal types. In this way, ideal types become real factors in community policy, planning and management. In fact, much of our law, policy and regulation is based on ideal principles; and deviations therefrom are considered to be improper, irrational and/or illegal. At the same time, there are those who suggest that behavior is not so much directed by goals and principles as by emotions and reactions to events as they occur. While we proceed with the plan of separating our discussion into two ideal types, the counterposition of ideal vs. actual, and rational vs. subjective will be a constant theme. We use the concept of ideal types to make a distinction between the two dominant paradigms, and then to extend their application to the realm of policy, planning and management.

The Consensus and Conflict Models of Society

Ralf Dahrendorf (1959) characterizes Western political thought as being dichotomized into two competing macro-views of society. According to **consensus theory,** social order results from a dominant set of shared values. People create communities to promote common interests and to escape from the "nasty, brutish and short" life of the precivilized. This perspective, in turn, leads to an **integration theory of society** which suggests that society is a relatively stable equilibrium based on a consensus of shared values and common patterns of interaction. **Systems theory** is associated with this perspective.

The competing paradigm, **conflict theory,** asserts that social order is based on domination and constraint. Communities result from a survival-of-the-fittest contest wherein the prize to the winners is the right to impose their will on others. This perspective, in turn, leads to a **coercion theory of society** wherein contending forces continually vie for domination and control. Dahrendorf identifies four tenets of each paradigm as follows:

CONSENSUS THEORY

> **Every society is a relatively persistent, stable structure of elements.**

> Every society is a well-integrated structure of elements.

> Every element in a society has a function, i.e., renders a contribution to its maintenance as a system.

> Every functioning social structure is based on a consensus of values among its members. (Dahrendorf, 1959, p. 161)

CONFLICT THEORY

> Every society is at every point subject to processes of change; social change is ubiquitous.

> Every society displays at every point dissensus and conflict; social conflict is ubiquitous.

> Every element in a society renders a contribution to its disintegration and change.

> Every society is based on the coercion of some of its members by others. (Dahrendorf, 1959, p. 162)

The theorist points out that these perspectives represent "two faces of society," and should be viewed as such. Each side focuses on certain aspects of the totality to explain certain phenomena. Consensus or systems theory asks why societies hang together, and conflict theory asks why they change. We might say that consensus theory tends to be more optimistic, looking at the positive side of society. By focusing on shared values, voluntary compliance, consensus, cooperation, and mutual benefit, society appears to be comprised of people who join together in a common venture. The results are integration, stability and equilibrium. The less rosy view of society observes that dissimilar interests and imbalances in power lead to the domination of some by others. This situation creates systems of stratification and hierarchy,whereby some individuals and groups can control others, and they extract greater portions of social goods--class, status, power--for themselves. The following table identifies major characteristics of the two approaches.

CONSENSUS THEORY	CONFLICT THEORY
Rationalist Perspective	Realist Perspective
Shared Values and Goals	Dissimilar Interests
Harmony	Cleavage
Man is Rational	Man is Irrational
Unity	Opposition
Consensus	Constraint
Voluntary Cooperation	Enforced Constraint
System	Hierarchy
Stability/Equilibrium	Change/Disequilibrium
Systems Persist	Systems Change
Cooperation	Conflict
Mutual Benefit	Status, Privilege
Integration	Stratification
Discretion	Control
Reinforces Existing Norms	Generates New Norms

It is important to recognize that at some point, each of these perspectives must confront the other. On the one hand, conflict occurs within some generalized structure of relationships--a system. And, on the other hand, systems would be immobilized, "dead," if there were no frictional interactions and movement of resources from some units to others. By being aware of both of these perspectives, we can approach the questions of change and stability with the understanding that each is but a "face" of the other. Reality reflects each face from the perspective of the viewer.

The Program Planning and Management Cycle

The model on the next page depicts the systemic relationships which should exist for an organization to effectively pursue its goals. As we consider the ideal characteristics of this model in the next few sections, keep the two perspectives of society in mind. If each unit does its job and interfaces perfectly with others, the organization will run effectively and efficiently. In reality, different actors often approach tasks with different values and goals, communication and interaction are not perfect, tasks are not always performed according to specifications, and schedules may not always be met. Moreover, the systems approach helps us to understand that slippage in one area will most likely lead to delays and problems in others. The designs and ideas generated at the conceptual policy research and planning stages are often out of synchronization with the empirical and experiential events which confront those units involved in implementation and operations. Additional conflict may also arise from professional rivalries and the hierarchical nature of formal organizations. These themes will accompany us throughout our consideration of several forms of planning, organization-implementation and management.

Programming: Four Major Functions

Four primary functions which are essential to the operation of community systems are:

1. **Program Planning.**

2. **Program Development and Implementation.**

3. **Program Operations.**

4. **Program Monitoring and Evaluation.**

These functions occur logically in this order as a policy emerges from idea to action, from planning to operations. Conceptualization and planning are prerequisite to testing and implementation; which, in turn, precede the actual delivery of services. In order to assure that services are meeting their objectives, operations must be tied closely to program monitoring and evaluation.

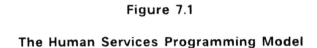

Figure 7.1

The Human Services Programming Model

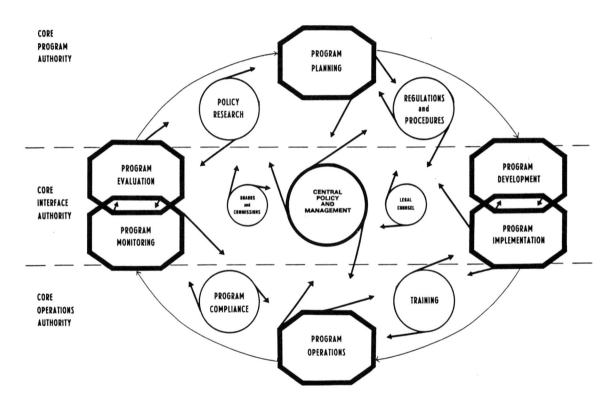

Four supportive or auxiliary functions are associated with the four primary functions. The auxiliary functions are:

A. Policy Research.

B. The Development of Regulations and Procedures.

C. Training and Staff Development.

D. Compliance.

These four auxiliary functions are important adjuncts to the primary functions. **Policy research** is directed to identifying options and mapping alternative approaches to carrying out policy. Formal articulation of **rules and regulations** to guide the implementation of programs provides legally binding and authoritative bases for action. **Training and staff development** promotes consistency and high quality performance of tasks by staff throughout the organization. And **compliance** activities are directed toward assurance that the terms of agreements are met and uniform application of policies occurs.

The Programming Process

The general programming process begins with identification of goals, and decisions on policy by those responsible for the direction of the organization--generally the top of the organizational hierarchy. The ideal-type process then moves through the following steps in a cyclical manner:

A. The consideration of alternative approaches to achieve the goals.

B. The design of means by which the chosen approach and the goals can be reached through the design of programs.

C. **The development of methods and tools for implementing programs.**

> **C(1). The writing and interpreting of rules and procedures to guide implementation of programs.**

D. **Testing, demonstrating, or piloting the programs.**

> **D(1). The provision of training to operations staff to assure knowledge and understanding of the new behaviors which are expected.**

E. **The actual implementation of the program community-wide, and continuing delivery of programs.**

> **E(1). Observation of compliance to assure that policies, regulations and procedures are implemented according to plan.**

F. **The monitoring and evaluation of programs to ascertain whether the delivery of services is in accordance with plans, and whether the programs are meeting objectives and goals as specified.**

This completes one "iteration" of the cycle. The process is then reiterated as evaluations inform policy research about areas remaining to be addressed and/or imperfections in existing programs. New strategies and alternative approaches are then designed either in response to evaluations by the organization, or in response to initiatives from outside sources.

Interactions Between Functions

Note the arrows on the chart. The arrows indicate areas of more intense interaction between functions. Thus, policy research receives direction from the central policy and management authorities, and it requires major inputs from both program evaluation and program planning. Training, on the other hand, is directly involved with program implementation and operations. The arrows are intended to indicate that sub-iterations may occur in any program or project cycle as problems occur or experience suggests that revisions may be in order.

It is also important to recognize that, in reality, action may **short-circuit,** or **shunt,** from one function to another. During the program development and implementation stages, for example, a plan may prove to be unworkable. Thus, a 'shunt' back to the planning stage may be required. Or, an evaluation may be performed during a pilot implementation which calls the basic goals into question-- leading to new policy research. Sometimes, too, officials may "jump the gun," so to speak by going directly from idea to operations without careful planning and development. It may be helpful to picture channels or spokes going from each function to all the others. This **"wheel"** model of the programming process was identified by Zietlow (1980) in a study of energy projects in Pennsylvania.

Note, too, that the model is divided horizontally into three general types of responsibility or "authority." In many organizations there is a general division of responsibility between those who attend primarily to goals and ideas, and those who implement and deliver. Sometimes these distinctions are made as **"staff,"** and **"line"** functions. Our model suggests that both complementary and conflictual relationships between **idea** and **action** tend to exist, and that there are general divisions between those who work on the question, "What should we be doing?" and the issue of "This is what we are doing."

>>Note the counter position of what might be seen as opposite functions on the chart. How is each function both a balance for and in conflict with its counterpart directly opposite on the chart? Note this relationship for both the primary and the auxiliary functions.<<

While idea and action are evident at all stages, there are some units which have as their "**core**" responsibility attention to policies, plans and regulations. We identify them as having "core program authority." Those who have primary responsibility for day-to-day program operations are labeled "core operations authority." And finally, idea and action must be brought together into a well-running organization. This "core interface authority" occurs as plans are brought to the development and implementation stage; and it occurs as program monitoring and evaluation provide comparisons of whether operations conform to the goals and plans of the organization. The next sections provide additional definition and explication of each of the stages of our general programming model.

The Eight Stages of the Policy and Programming Model

Central Policy and Management: The central policy and management role is generally performed by an agency head, or by an executive board or planning council for a multiagency body. Overall responsibility for both internal policy and performance rests here. Actors responsible for this function generally also handle relationships with the interorganizational environment--other organizations and subsystems in the community.

Those responsible for this function examine major issues, priorities and proposals. Decisions on the issues and problems that will be addressed by the organization are made here. All units are ultimately answerable to this function.

Policy Research: Policy research is concerned with "mapping alternative approaches to a problem or issue and with specifying potential differences in the intention, effect, and cost of various programs." (Etzioni, 1971) It deals with formulating strategies to deal with the fundamental problems and goals of the organization. It is concerned with values and purposes, and attempts to "clarify goals and the relations among them, as well as among goals and sets of means." Policy research is thus critical in nature. This is the place where the most "pure" ideas can be aired and considered for their potentiality and feasibility.

Program Planning: Program planning, when compared to policy research, is technical and instrumental. It deals with "designing means by which goals may be achieved." (Young, 1966) Planning involves the design of programs and technology to implement policy and program decisions. The task of the planners is to prepare a set of specifications which is capable of being implemented. In many organizations, the policy research, planning and program development functions are carried out by the same staff.

Regulations and Procedures: Plans must be translated into written rules and procedures to guide workers. This is an auxiliary function wherein existing and proposed rules are considered and interrelated. The legality of plans is tested at this stage. Manuals of regulations and guidelines for operation, developed at this stage, provide the basis for implementation and action. The feasibility of plans is frequently examined here, often suggesting the need for further design or redesign.

Program Development/Implementation: One step beyond planning, program development is concerned with testing and preparing for implementation. This function involves the development of new program modules, new activities and new methods of delivering services in response to the requirements of long- and short-range plans. The coordination of experimental and demonstration projects, and their relationship with the broader community are addressed here. The "nitty-gritty" issues of transforming a plan into a program are confronted in the development and implementation stages. It is at this point that the interface between the planning/design and operations aspects of an organization occurs. Piloting, demonstration and/or experimentation provide for reality testing prior to general implementation in the field.

Training and Staff Development: Training is concerned with developing the necessary capabilities--that is, knowledge, skills, and abilities--to ensure that programs can be carried out effectively. It involves the development, planning and implementation of training programs, institutes, seminars, workshops, and courses for professional and technical employees. The training function also includes coordination of varied agency training activities and the development, promotion, and implementation of broad agency or interagency training policies. Training units typically also provide consultation to other units and assessments of training needs.

A two-way relationship exists between this auxiliary function and the primary functions of program development/implementation and program operations. Training receives inputs from the former in terms of the type of knowledge, skills, or abilities which are required. In turn, it takes action to impart the required knowledge, skills, and abilities to operations staff.

Program Operations and Service Delivery: The delivery of programs and/or services falls under the general rubric of "program operations." The specific content of program operations varies from system to system. The delivery of health, justice, social services, nutrition, income maintenance, and services to youth and the aged are direct services in most American communities. The regulation and control of housing, transportation, recreation and cultural functions, and community infrastructure all have operational aspects to be considered. Since our purpose is to examine the policy and planning aspects of community systems in general, we will not deal directly with specific systems here. Most importantly, however, the content and potentialities of any policy, plan or design may be severely constrained by the nature of the current program operations of a particular subsystem. We do wish to point out two primary types of activity which are associated with program operations.

Maintenance Operations involve support for basic administrative activities which are necessary for any ongoing program. The activities of budgeting, personnel administration, record-keeping, equipment and supply, and other logistical support fall under this rubric.

Service Operations involves the supervision and management of the organization's service product. The professional and technical staff who deliver services and regulate community systems fall under this rubric.

Miringoff (1980) distinguishes between these two types of managerial activities by pointing out differences between the maintenance activities and the service activities of operations staff. Maintenance activities are essential to organizational survival; however, service activities determine the quality of goal achievement --organizational output. Attention to the latter is particularly important in monitoring and evaluation activities.

Compliance: The compliance function involves investigative and audit activities which are directed to assuring that the letter of the law, including regulations and procedures, is kept. The uniform application of written policies, regulations and procedures provide guides by which to compare actual operations. This "policing" function is intended to assure proper operation of all system units, supervision and issuance of permits and licenses, and maintenance of overall quality control.

Program Monitoring and Evaluation: These two related functions provide the interface between operations and planning, and between compliance and policy research. Program monitoring focuses more on assessing the short-term activities of organizational units, while program evaluation focuses on goals and longer-range impact. These assessment functions involve a process of information gathering which allows decisions to be made on the efficiency and effectiveness of the overall system and its subunits. The purpose of these functions is to identify, explain and record areas of success and failure of the organization in order that future actions can be planned accordingly.

The program monitoring function also provides feedback to the compliance and operations units in the form of technical assistance and analyses. Similarly, the evaluation function provides information for the policy and planning units to allow reconsideration and redirection as appropriate. Finally, these functions signal the end of one cycle and the beginning of another. Thus, evaluation generates policy research, and the cycle continues.

The Programming Model and the Organizational Hierarchy

The programming model explicated above is based on an ideal-type conceptualization of the functions that are necessary for a community program or subsystem to operate. We have noted the reality of short-circuits, or shunts, and that disagreements, discontinuities and/or conflicts may develop between functions. The fact that formal organizations tend to be organized in a hieirarchy of authority lends additional "irrationality" to the process.

The next two pages provide a real-life illustration of how our model might apply to an existing organization. Figure 7.1 presents an organizational chart for a "Department of Human Services." While based on a state-level department, this **"table of organization"** could apply to a county, city, or metropolitan area as well. Most organization charts depict all offices in a descending hierarchy from the top official--in this case the "Secretary." Thus, the **"chain of command"** is made clear, and each unit knows its hierarchical authority relationship to others. For example, the directors of offices, bureaus, or deputy secretaries, would generally have equal authority to their counterparts, but over different aspects of organizational activities. We have arranged this chart to depict the different "core" authorities as identified on the programming model. The usual organization chart would depict the "core program authority" offices as being below the "Secretary."

Figure 7.3 depicts the offices on the table of organization as they relate to the functions on our programming model. Note that several units are typically involved in each of the functions. Note, too, that some units have responsibilities for several functions. Thus, the Office of Inter-Program Planning and Evaluation has responsibilities for policy research, program planning, and both interface functions. Likewise, the different program offices have policy research and planning units. The need to coordinate and to interrelate these various units becomes a major task in modern organizations.

In our polycentric system, neither are the program functions performed as a totally consensual process, nor does conflict reign supreme. Rather, elements of both are infused throughout decisionmaking and action. The next section will present dual

244

Figure 7.2

Organization of the Department
of Human Services

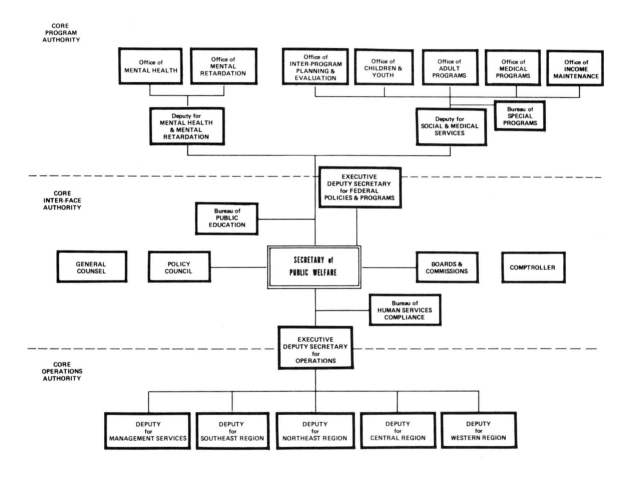

Figure 7.3

Structure and Functional
Interrelationships

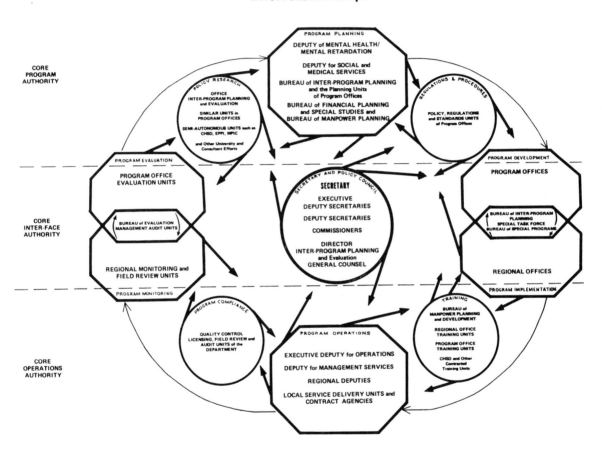

CORE
PROGRAM
AUTHORITY

CORE
INTER-FACE
AUTHORITY

CORE
OPERATIONS
AUTHORITY

PROGRAM PLANNING

DEPUTY of MENTAL HEALTH/
MENTAL RETARDATION

DEPUTY for SOCIAL and
MEDICAL SERVICES

BUREAU of INTER-PROGRAM PLANNING
and the Planning Units
of Program Offices

BUREAU of FINANCIAL PLANNING
and SPECIAL STUDIES and
BUREAU of MANPOWER PLANNING

POLICY RESEARCH

OFFICE
INTER-PROGRAM PLANNING
and EVALUATION

SIMILAR UNITS in
PROGRAM OFFICES

SEMI-AUTONOMOUS UNITS such as
CHSD, EPPI, WPIC

and Other University and
Consultant Efforts

REGULATIONS & PROCEDURES

POLICY, REGULATIONS
and STANDARDS UNITS
of Program Offices

PROGRAM EVALUATION

PROGRAM OFFICE
EVALUATION UNITS

BUREAU of EVALUATION
MANAGEMENT AUDIT UNITS

REGIONAL MONITORING and
FIELD REVIEW UNITS

PROGRAM MONITORING

SECRETARY AND POLICY COUNCIL

SECRETARY

EXECUTIVE
DEPUTY SECRETARIES

DEPUTY SECRETARIES

COMMISSIONERS

DIRECTOR
INTER-PROGRAM PLANNING
and Evaluation
GENERAL COUNSEL

PROGRAM DEVELOPMENT

PROGRAM OFFICES

BUREAU of INTER-PROGRAM
PLANNING
SPECIAL TASK FORCE
BUREAU of SPECIAL PROGRAMS

REGIONAL OFFICES

PROGRAM IMPLEMENTATION

PROGRAM COMPLIANCE

QUALITY CONTROL
LICENSING, FIELD REVIEW and
AUDIT UNITS of the
DEPARTMENT

PROGRAM OPERATIONS

EXECUTIVE DEPUTY for OPERATIONS

DEPUTY for MANAGEMENT SERVICES

REGIONAL DEPUTIES

LOCAL SERVICE DELIVERY UNITS and
CONTRACT AGENCIES

TRAINING

BUREAU of
MANPOWER PLANNING
and DEVELOPMENT

REGIONAL OFFICE
TRAINING UNITS

PROGRAM OFFICE
TRAINING UNITS

CHSD and Other
Contracted
Training Units

perspectives on policymaking and analysis. Throughout the discussion it will become clear that we are dealing with highly complex and intricate processes. Change does not occur without effort. It will also be apparent that change does not come about by either chance or the design of some evil (or benign) genius. Change occurs as a result of individuals and groups working through community structures.

Consensus and Conflict Approaches to Policy and Analysis

The consensus and conflict paradigms are not restricted to theories of society. They have been incorporated and elaborated in a variety of approaches to analysis and change. At the most general level, John P. van Gigch has articulated two methodologies of change; and applications in policymaking are postulated by Charles E. Lindblom. (van Gigch, 1974; Lindblom, 1959) While not totally parallel to the two dominant paradigms, there is enough correspondence to suggest parallel discussion here as ideal types.

Lindblom identifies two approaches to policy formulation. One approach, the **"rational-deductive,"** is **theory-based.** A systematic process of goal-setting, identification of values and comparison of alternative strategies of action leads to a conscious decision to act. It begins with specified ends, generally those given by the hierarchy, and seeks the most efficent means thereto. This approach stresses highly quantitative analysis to identify the costs and benefits of each alternative. After long-range, comprehensive analysis of this sort, a decision is made which maximizes the benefits for the least cost. This approach is goal-oriented, viewing "good" as the most cost-beneficial option.

Another approach, which Lindblom calls **"limited successive approximations,"** or "muddling through," is means (rather than goal-oriented). It emphasises the **process** of politics as an interactional field between actors with different goals: thus, goals cannot be specified with precision. With this approach, the policymaker selects an objective in a general way, and then takes small steps in that direction. Thus, the policymaker may make tentative steps in one direction, be thwarted, and then move in another--perhaps even shifting the objective in response to environmental events.

This approach seeks to build from the current situation by small degrees. Viable policy options are those which are in vogue with powerful interests. Data and analysis are used to support one's position, and less so as a way to identify possible directions, or to provide definitive data on which to base decisions. This approach is **interest-oriented,** viewing "good" as the outcome of contending forces in the political process.

Van Gigch's two methodologies of change, **systems improvement** and **systems design,** provide additional insight into alternative approaches. The "systems improvement" approach takes the goals of a system as given. It then seeks to use rational-deductive analysis to identify problems, and to design means to bring the system back into compliance with given norms. Thus, systems improvement looks inward, using rational-analytic methods to improve the existing system. It can thus be said to contribute to maintaining the equilibrium of the larger system within which it operates.

The "systems design" approach, on the other hand, looks outward, asking how the focal system fits into the broader system of which it is a part. The extrospective outlook is thus open to consideration of changes in purpose and goals--and in turn to change of the system itself. Thus, the "problem" is defined in relation to its role in the entire interorganizational or intersystem field, asking what goals and actions are appropriate to a changing environment. The systems design approach is most compatible with moving in limited successive approximations toward some general long-range goal. One would expect that sophisticated policymakers and managers, however, would use whatever technical and analytic tools are at hand to enhance their understanding of both subsystem and environmental events. This would be done in full recognition of the complexity of the broader system and the shifting nature of community systems. Analysis, in this frame of reference, is a tool to aid in gathering data for decisions, rather than a definitive way to secure answers on what is "good." The following chart lists the major characteristics of the consensus and conflict approaches to policy and change.

CONSENSUS-ORIENTED	CONFLICT-ORIENTED
Systems Improvement	Systems Design
Comprehensive Planning	Successive Approximations
Builds from Theory	Builds from Current Policy
Cost-Benefit Analysis	Assess Community Interests
Goal/Ends-Oriented	Process/Means Oriented
Make This System Work	Adapt to the Broader System
System-Inward Focus	System-Outward Focus
Objective-Deductive	Subjective-Inductive
Long-Range Calculations	Short-Range Calculations
Idealist	Realist

The identification of these different perspectives allows us to choose more explicitly our role in the policy process. They help us to understand some of the latent conservatism of the quantifiers and technicians, as well as the apparent radicalism of those who focus on the clashing of interests. The next chapter extends our understanding of these strains to the planning, organizing-implementation, and management of community systems.

Chapter VII

REFERENCES

Dahrendorf, Ralf. **Class and Class Conflict in Industrial Society.** Stanford, Calif: Stanford University Press, 1959, esp. Ch. V.

Etzioni, Amitai. "Policy Research," **The American Sociologist,** 6, Supplementary Issue, June 1971, p. 8.

Gates, Bruce L. **Social Program Administration.** Englewood Cliffs, N. J.: Prentice-Hall, 1980.

Lindblom, Charles E. "The Science of Muddling Through," **Public Administration Review,** 29, Spring 1959, 79-88.

Miringoff, Marc L. **Management in Human Service Organizations.** N. Y.: MacMillan, 1980.

van Gigch, John. **Applied General Systems Theory.** N. Y.: Harper and Row, 1974.

Weber, Max. **The Theory of Social and Economic Organization,** ed., Talcott Parsons. N. Y.: Oxford University Press, 1947, Free Press Paperback, 1964.

Young, Robert C. "Goals and Goal-Setting," **Journal of the American Institute of Planners,** 23, March 1969, 76-85.

Zietlow, Carl P. **Action Research Applied to Community Development, Local Governments and Energy Conservation.** University Park, Pa.: The Pennsylvania State University, Ph.D. Thesis in Community Systems Planning and Development, 1980.

Chapter VIII

PLANNING AND MANAGING COMMUNITY
COMMUNITY SYSTEMS II: SIX MODELS
OF COMMUNITY ENGAGEMENT

"The means-and-end moralists or non-doers
always wind up on their ends without any means."
                                        -Saul Alinsky
                                    "Of Means and Ends"

"If you don't know where you want to go, any path
will take you."

                                        -Alice
                                    "Alice in Wonderland"

To What End "Change"?

"Does the end justify the means?" This question perennially confronts the theory and practice of community systems. On the one hand, there are those who argue that ethical, lasting change can be brought about only through democratic processes, rational discussion, and careful consideration of all groups and factors involved. Change, it is argued, should occur through existing community structures without resort to violence or harm to any of the parties involved. Only peaceful, considerate, deliberative means can produce lasting, legitimate ends. On the other hand, there are others who point to the lessons of the past and argue that those in positions of power and influence (i.e., the "power structure") will always control the political process and resist change. An "Iron Law of Oligarchy" teaches us that other means are often necessary to correct inequities, injustices, and imbalances of power.* The end or goal is really the supreme object to be sought, so whatever means are available should be used.

The solution to this dilemma is neither simple nor clear-cut, as we look at our history in the United States. Fundamental documents of the American Revolution, for example, embrace each position. The Declaration of Independence is not only a statement of human rights; it is also a strong declaration that violent means are often necessary to reach a just political end. The violent conflict which led to the establishment of the United States is celebrated every Fourth of July as a victory for freedom and self-determination. Our Constitution, however, sets out very definite and limited processes for the control and exercise of power and authority. Our country has both the longest peaceful democratic government in history and it has been confronted by "other means" of change in practically every generation. The Boston Tea Party, the Civil War, the labor movement, women's suffrage, the "Red Scare," the Civil Rights Movement, the "War on Poverty," the anti-Vietnam War peace movement, and the recent antinuclear movement have all been accompanied by "other" means of demonstration and protest. On a worldwide basis, we observe stability being maintained by both democratic and repressive regimes. Instability occurs both as peoples and groups seek to establish major reforms or revolutionary systems and when military dictators take over democratic regimes. Conflicts are manifest daily in the form of violent opposition movements, terrorism, and protests as means directed to achieve social and political change.

Does a valued end justify any means? Alinsky's answer is to restate the question. "Does this **particular** end justify this **particular** means?" (Alinsky, 1971) And, "where you stand depends on where you sit." Again, the response does not give us the easy out of justifying one approach or the other; rather it imposes a requirement to examine both means and ends, and then to take **personal responsibility** for our actions.

----

* Michels suggests that anywhere a hierarchy exists, there will be a tendency for those in power to rule in their own interests--hence the "iron law" that an oligarchy will result.

The debate over means-ends ethics complements our consideration of ideal types of society and approaches to community systems. And it extends our discussion to the realm of strategies of practice. The consensus model and related approaches to change are generally associated with the cooperative, work-within-the-system side of the debate: only approved means are legitimate. The conflict model is associated more with the "ends justifies the means" position. Different strategies of change emanate from, and are often rationalized by, proponents of each.

This chapter explores six approaches, or **strategies,** to directing and changing community systems and human services programs. Our discussion of strategies is based first on the principle developed in previous chapters that policies establish goals and general directions--the "ends" of community systems. We have also established that fundamental social paradigms provide approaches to observation and analysis, as well as to how change should be brought about--the "means" of community action. Synthesis of our knowledge of policies, systems, and approaches to knowledge leads us to consider the means-ends dilemma in the design of strategies for engaging in actions to maintain, to reform, to eliminate, or to radically change programs or organizations. Consideration of ideal types of planning, organizing-implementation, and management in this chapter will provide a repertoire of options with which to approach the development and operation of community systems.

A Note On Strategy, Tactics, and Skills

Before presenting the six models of engagement, a note on the meaning of "strategy" is appropriate. **"Strategy"** is generally viewed as the most general, long-term approach to an action situation, and can be compared to **"tactics,"** which is more immediate and short-term. "Strategy" is **extrospective,** based on total system considerations. "Tactics" is **introspective,** directed to the interaction of subunits within a system. Strategy is an attempt to select the "best" course of action in light of the actions of other actors and assessment of their anticipated actions. Tactics involve the way an actor deploys its resources toward implementation of a broader strategy. Thus, strategy involves decisions about the desired goals and the actions to be taken toward **both** means and ends: the desired goals and the actions to be taken toward their achievement. Tactics involves management of the organization or group according to the means (i. e., strategy) selected.

Skill refers to the capabilities of individual units or actors. Skill involves the development of expertise, ability or proficiency at a particular task or craft, and is, therefore, more specific and limited than either strategy or tactics. Strategy and tactics are **interactive** concepts. Skill is not. Although skills establish a level of competence and readiness for interactional events, an individual can develop and exercise skills without reference to other actors.

>>Consider athletic competition. One can develop skill in shooting basketballs, weightlifting, running, pole-vaulting, fly-casting, etc., without reference to others. When involved in application or competition, however, strategy and tactics come into play to determine how the skills will be applied in an interactional situation.

In community systems, police may have a strategy of reacting to crimes, or of active prevention. Health can be addressed through immunizations, nutrition, exercise; or by treatment after illness occurs. Mental health can employ a hospital-based "warehousing" strategy, or a community-based "normalization" approach. Consider the implications of each of these alternative strategies for the residents of the community, the differences in tactics which would be involved, and the skills required.<<

Skills are important in establishing the probability that individual units or actors will be able to perform the tasks required by tactics, which in turn are the basis for the implementation of strategy. Each of these three levels can be said to deal with a different level or subsystem of the broader system.

Skills = The capability of individual units or subsystems to perform specific tasks.

Tactics = The arrangement and interaction of units or subsystems in a concerted action.

Strategy = The direction chosen for a system in an interactional engagement with other systems.

Consider, for example, two organizations in the hospitality industry. Each has the goal of establishing a successful organization and making a profit selling hamburgers near a busy airport. "Boffo Burgers" develops a strategy of giving high-quality, nutritious burgers in a sophisticated, relaxed setting. Tactical concerns which flow from this decision require a chef and staff with excellent skills, waiters and waitresses trained in quality service skills, a generous selection on the menu, and an expensive physical plant. "Speedo Beefo," the competitor, has a strategy of providing inexpensive, fast food. Its tactics call for limited choice, staff trained in speed rather than quality service, less expensive cuts of meat (fillers in the beef), and a cheap but clean physical plant.

If the environment in which these two establishments operate is such that customers are generally in a hurry to get to their next plane or destination, then we would expect the "Speedo Beefo" organization to be more successful. This example points out the importance of recognizing that strategic decisions must be made in consideration of environmental conditions and other actors. It is likely that those in charge of Boffo Burgers have misread its marketing environment and made poor strategic choices. The consequence of such poor strategic planning and decisionmaking is that tactical choices do not turn out to be good investments. In effect, the "superior" tactics and skills of the Boffo Burgers operation are destined for failure in this particular scenario.

The choice of strategy is thus a key decision in the action process. It sets the overall direction for a system, and determines which tactics and skills are appropriate in a specific situation. In the sections which follow, we will examine six ideal-type options for community engagement and action. These **models** parallel the primary functions of our general programming model. **Planning** is addressed to problem identification, evaluation, and the design of programs for change; **organizing-implementation** is concerned with how a plan takes shape and is manifest in community programs and organizations; and **management** provides the direction, control and administrative aspect of ongoing operations. Also remember that although the choice of strategies for engaging community organizations, groups, and programs in ongoing action and change is seldom clear-cut, the actions taken will have definite impact on the future. **(Not to decide is to decide.)** We now proceed to the explication of two ideal-type models of each of these three general areas. As we examine these models, it is important to keep in mind the fundamental principles of systems and how community systems are organized in the United States, the two dominant paradigms of social philosophy and policymaking, and the need to make action decisions on the means-ends question.

Two Models of Planning

Planning generally refers to formulation of ideas and/or actions into a scheme to accomplish some purpose or objective. Planning is **proactive** in considering anticipated future actions. It is **directive** in setting out a proposed course of action. And it is a **process** designed to provide for the selection from optional possible directions. Planning should lead first to the selection of a **strategy** to reach the goals of a system or program based on an assessment of **environmental conditions** and **system capabilities**. Then **tactics** can be considered, and requisite skills developed. Consider the following definitions of planning:

. . . a social process for reaching a rational decision.
                                        –Robert A. Dahl

"Planning is the design of a desired future and of effective ways of bringing it about."
                                        –Russell L. Ackoff

PLANNING IS THE PROCESS OF PREPARING A SET OF DECISIONS FOR ACTION DIRECTED AT ACHIEVING GOALS BY PREFERABLE MEANS.
                                        –Yehezkel Dror

A **plan** is a course of action which can be carried into effect, which can be expected to lead to the attainment of the ends sought, and which someone (an effectuating organization) intends to carry into effect. (By contrast, a course of action which could not be carried out, which would not have the consequences intended, or which no one intends to carry out is a "utopian scheme" rather than a plan.)
                                        –Edward Banfield

. . . by definition, planning is a comprehensive and rational process.
                                        –Ruth Glass

"Speaking generally, planning is deciding in advance what is to be done; that is, a plan is a projected course of action.
                                        –William H. Newman

. . . plans are proposals of concerted action to achieve goals.
                                        –Alan Altshuler

A PLAN IS A PROACTIVE LOOK AT THE PRESENT.
                                        –Hyman and Miller

Planning thus asks, "How can we get to future state 'Y' from the present 'X'?" It emphasizes a rational-technical process of problem identification, data gathering and analysis, assessment of options, and evaluation.

Ideal Types: Traditional Planning and Advocacy Planning*

The planning process described above sounds highly rational and comprehensive. We all know, however, that many, perhaps most, plans are not comprehensive, and rationality is a relative concept. Moreover, our earlier discussion of ideal-type models of policy identified both "rationalist" and "realist" perspectives. These two perspectives carry through to the planning process as well. Planning may vary from a consensus-oriented, highly technical and rational process with full use of computer technology, mathematical models and cost-benefit analysis, to conflict-oriented, interest-driven planning based on experiential data-gathering and intuitive analysis. Two models of planning which reflect these approaches have been identified in the literature as "traditional planning" and "advocacy planning." (Stockdale, 1976)

Figure 8.2 presents the primary characteristics of the two ideal-type models of planning. **Traditional planning** conforms most closely to the idealist rational-comprehensive model of policy, and thus is associated with the consensus model of society. It emphasizes broad goals related to the overall community and seeks to address substantive social problems--health, housing, justice, nutrition, etc. A community-wide plan for recreation or health based on an overall assessment of needs and problems would be typical. Traditional planning is based on the premise that our highly complex and technological postindustrial society requires technical experts to design and to anticipate the future.

----

* For further information see Stockdale's elaboration of Rothman's strategies of community organization which provides the conceptual underpinnings for these models. (Stockdale, 1976)

Figure 8.2

Two Models of Community Planning

PRACTICE VARIABLES	TRADITIONAL PLANNING	ADVOCACY PLANNING
Goal Categories of Community Action.	Problem-solving with regard to broad, substantive community problems (task goals).	Problem-solving with regard to sub-community problems, shifting of resources (task or process goals).
Assumptions Concerning Community Structure and Problem Conditions.	Substantive overall social problems: health, housing, transportation,etc.	Disadvantaged populations, social injustice, inequity, unserved segments in social problem areas.
Basic Change Strategy	Needs analysis and rational-technical program design for the overall community.	Needs analysis and rational-technical program design to represent interests of a segment or sub-population.
Characteristic Change Tactics and Techniques.	Consensus. Rational presenation of "facts."	Campaign or contest. Interest-oriented presentation of facts.
Salient Practitioner Roles.	Fact-gatherer and analyst, program implementer, facilitator.	Fact-gatherer and analyst, plus organizer, advocate, partisan.
Medium of Change	Manipulation of data and formal organizations.	Manipulation of data and program support by client population.
Orientation Toward Power Structure.	Subordinant: power structure as employers and sponsors.	Engagement: power structure as target for action.
Boundary of Constituency or Client System.	Total geographic community, or sub-system as consumers or recipients.	Community segment-- attempts to co-opt power structure to client goals.
Assumptions Regarding Interests of Community Sub-Parts.	Common interests, or reconcilable differences.	Conflicting interests which are not easily reconcilable; scarce resources.

*Adapted from Stockdale's elaboration of a typology developed initially by Rothman. (Stockdale, 1976; Rothman, 1974)

The contrasting approach, **advocacy planning,** also utilizes technical skills and leadership, but focuses on subcommunity problems--neighborhoods, disadvantaged populations, unserved or underserved segments of the community. Problem-solving is directed to reallocation of resources toward a particular segment or program area. Fact-gathering and analysis are fundamental, and are employed from an activist-advocate perspective. Advocacy planning would thus work for improved recreation, health care, nutrition, or community control of police, for example, in a particular neighborhood or for a subgroup in the broader community.

Both types of planning tend to employ rational-technical technologies, to perform **task** goals, but from different community perspectives--the overall community or a subcommunity segment respectively. Advocacy planning, moreover, frequently employs process skills to mobilize affected citizens for support or implementation. The advocacy planner sees the power structure as a target for action; thus, there is a need to develop a power base for campaign or contest interactions with the authorities. Traditional planning, on the other hand, typically occurs within the power structure and is thus characterized by consensus tactics and rational presentation of "facts."

Planners of both types emphasize needs analysis, fact gathering, identification and evaluation of options and the design of programs and systems. "Let's get the facts and make a rational decision." Traditional planning emphasizes the preparation and presentation of the plan itself. Advocacy planning must focus not only on the plan, but the process of support for and acceptance of the plan by authorities. The former tends to assume that the plan will speak for itself; the latter must be an advocate for and partisan of the plan on behalf of the client group. Traditional planning views the plan as the end product to a much greater extent than advocacy planning, which views the plan as a means to the end of redistribution of resources.

Traditional planning is most closely associated with the consensus model of society, and thus relies on the existing power structure for support and implementation. Advocacy planning, in that it addresses community subgroups or segments, is in a conflict position, and thus requires campaign or contest tactics. The conflict model of society thus provides the more appropriate perspective for the advocacy planner.

It follows then that traditional planners are typically part of the overall community power structure. They are part of the 'machinery' of the authorities. Thus, they are in a **subordinate** relationship with the power structure. Advocacy planners, conversely, are typically part of an organization or subsystem which sees the overall power structure as a target of action. They are in a position which requires **engagement** of the authorities as a target for action. Thus, traditional planners are specialists of the power structure; and advocacy planners are specialists dedicated to change of the power structure.

The former perspective tends to assume a variable sum game (expanding resource base), while the latter views the political process as a zero sum game where the benefit of one party is usually at the expense of another. The traditional planner assumes that, if the overall system is taken care of in a carefully planned, rational manner, then the parts will be taken care of as well. The advocacy planner presumes that competing interests will contend in the arena of action, and that the disadvantaged can influence the distrubution of existing (scarce) resources if they are afforded the technical skills of planning. (Stockdale, 1976; Rothman, 1974)

Planning In Perspective

Planning occurs in all types of community organizations: police departments, welfare programs, mental health centers, hospitals, housing departments and transportation services all plan their activities in some manner. As understood in the profession, planning is a rational-technical process which is proactively directed to the design of strategy and tactics for the near- or long-term future. Planning should be distinguished from **utopian schemes,** which are unrealistic and would not meet intended goals, and from **reactive decisions,** which are simply on-the-spot responses to environmental events. While plans may have elements of each of these latter concepts (since it may not be possible to test ideas beforehand and quick responses to a changing environment are often necessary), the intent of the planner is to be proactive and rational in the choice of action.

Advocacy planning and traditional planning can be said to represent opposite ends of the planning continuum. A realistic plan will most likely have elements of both. Plans which have been incubated in a city planning department for a year or more, however, may be completely unfamiliar to both community decisionmakers and citizens. Hence there is often a need for the traditional planner to convince others of the feasibility and viability of the proposed course of action. Likewise, advocacy planners may find it useful to present data on how the overall community will benefit from her/his proposal. The development of support for implementation of a plan is crucial for a plan "to come together." The next section addresses approaches to the engineering of consent for implementing plans and policies.

Two Models of Organizing and Implementation

"The best laid plans of mice and men . . .," so the story goes, do not come to fruition because of unrealistic approaches to action. The cartoon on the next page depicts a popular view of planning. Our view is that many excellent plans frequently end up "on the shelf" because inadequate attention is given to the process of implementation. All too frequently, decisionmakers follow the decision to implement a plan with a directive to the operations or field staff to put it into effect. Such action is typically an ironclad prescription for failure. The process of translating the ideas and techniques specified in an "ivory tower" plan into action in the field is the most critical stage of organizational change; and it is the least understood and least anticipated in many situations.

Gerald Caiden refers to implementation as "The Achilles Heel of Administrative Reform."

> The evidence suggests that while ideas and proposals are legion, it is difficult to get anyone to do something about them. . . . Reform fails mainly at the implementation stage. . . . The reasons are fairly straightforward. The reformers remain outsiders to the situations they are trying to improve. (Caiden, 1976)

COMPREHENSIVE PLANNING

As Planners requested it

As the Director ordered it

As Engineering designed it

As ECO-Industries built it

As Providers corrected it

What the consumers wanted

The cartoon on this page was "lifted" from the Muncy Luminary, with the connivance of editor Bob Wilt. He said he in turn liberated it from the Windsor, Colo. Beacon, whose editor picked it up from the Greenville (Ala.) Advocate. Evidently it originated in a publication called the Montana Environmentalist. A good idea goes a long way, it seems. We thought readers would enjoy it.

The implementation of plans requires primary attention not only to the logic or technical quality of the plan, but also to the people and organizations that will be affected. That is, the plan is but a design for change; change is brought about only through the conviction and action of community actors. To get a feel for the dynamics of this engagement process, we draw upon the experience of two related fields which have a history of community action--community development and community organizing.

Community development is an international movement with roots in colonialism and religious evangelism. Its professional ties are to the fields of education and social work as applied to the developing areas. The U. N. Special Study on Social Conditions in Non-Self-Governing Territories in 1956 stated that "The concept of community development originated in the search for a program to compensate for the limitations of the conventional school system, and to enable education to provide for the progressive evolution of the peoples." (United Nations, 1956) This approach sought to promote the advancement of communities through educational and group processes directed to learning democracy. The goal was self-help, local initiative and local responsibility.

In the United States, these processes were applied first to rural areas. An extensive network of agricultural extension services was developed, and continues to serve through university and county programs. In urban areas, a social work process evolved from group work as **"community organizing."** Community organizing is rooted in the cooperative educational model of community development, and the early practice in urban areas emphasized self-help and collaborative strategies. Neighborhood workers, settlement houses, YMCA's, and group workers emphasized local involvement to solve local problems. In the decades of the 1950's and 1960's, however, discrimination, poverty and neglect of basic rights led to the emergence of confrontational approaches. Community organizers became involved in social movements, radical groups in the professions, and social justice.

The experience and practice of community development and community organizing are similar to those required for implementation, for they address the **process** of emplacing new or revised programs or systems in communities. This perspective is based on the fact that it is necessary for those wishing to implement a program or reform **(1) to gain the acceptance of those affected,**

(2) to gain access to those with influence over those affected, or (3) to acquire positions of power and influence themselves.

Implementation involves **setting a program in motion or in place.** Running and maintaining the organization on an ongoing basis are something else--control or management (addressed in the next section). Consider some statements from the literature about the fields of community development and organizing.

> "It is the hard next step after the decision, involving efforts to put in place--to make operational--what has been decided. . . . That is the stage in the policy process where so much can go wrong."
>
> –Walter Williams

> . . . **development of capacity to manage one's own (the individual, group, or community) life, ability to function as an integrated unit.**
>
> –Murray Ross

> The process of stimulating and assisting the local community to evaluate, plan, and coordinate its efforts.
>
> –Charles Zastrow

> TO FURNISH A WORKING RELATIONSHIP BETWEEN THE DEMOCRATIC PROCESS AND SPECIALISM.
>
> –Eduard C. Lindeman

> "The techniques of community organization encompass activities devoted to exchanging ideas, meeting, negotiating, bargaining, educating, accommodating, and on occasion, using authority and pressure."
>
> –Floyd Hunter et al.

> **It is concerned with the interrelationships of groups within communities, their integration and coordination in the interest of efficiency and unity of action.**
>
> –Jesse F. Steiner

THE TRANSFORMATION OF A PLAN FROM IDEA TO ACTION.

-Hyman and Miller

Implementation is that crucial phase of any program or system where a decision on a plan is made manifest in community life or it falls by the wayside ("ends up on the shelf"). Planners tend to be **"office-bound,"** dealing with facts, ideas and designs. Hopefully, they have plumbed the communities or groups for which they have planned so that the designs are realistic and feasible. Nevertheless, the process of moving from idea to reality is extended and complex. The orchestration of all aspects of system operations, including retraining existing staff, testing new technologies in the field, educating clients and consumers to a changed system, revising regulations and procedures, and myriad other details--
often while the existing system continues--is a serious undertaking. Implementation must be **"community-bound,"** or **"people-bound,"** concerned with the interrelationships of new or revised programs to existing organizations and groups at the community or delivery level. It must provide for the integration and coordination of new technologies and new procedures. It must gain the support of both the people and the leaders. And this transformation must be done efficiently and effectively. Implementation must confront the activities of an ongoing community system to achieve a particular set of new or revised goals. Implementation thus attends to the **means** by which new **ends** are achieved.

Ideal Types: Locality Development and Social Action*

Community development and community organization are rooted in the consensus-oriented, self-help and education approaches to change. The articulation of conflict-oriented

----

For further information, see Rothman's (1974) article on community organization strategies, which provides the conceptual base for this section.

approaches in the mid-20th century to deal with racial discrimination, urban poverty and exclusion of many citizens from realization of "The American Dream," led to the emergence of confrontational approaches to change. As noted earlier, "other means" are not unknown in America; however, previous experience tended to spring from grassroots action and was based in voluntary action. The adoption of conflict approaches by professionals signified a change in the level at which the organizing and leadership for confrontation might occur. These events in the U.S. were not without parallels elsewhere. Internationally, the decline of colonialism was attended by a "revolution of rising expectations." Nationalist movements and separatist groups frequently used coercive approaches to confront their masters. Mohandas Ghandi is well known for his nonviolent strategies of passive resistance and civil disobedience. "Liberation" movements in Algeria, Viet Nam, and Cuba provide examples of violent confrontational approaches. And the Industrial Areas Foundation of Saul Alinsky provided one significant source for articulating conflict-oriented approaches and for training organizers in the United States. While we are concerned most directly with the implementation of planned change in local communities, the national and international movements give evidence of the efficacy of both conflict and consensus approaches to change. Two models of grassroots action which reflect these approaches have been articulated by Rothman in the literature as "locality development" and "social action."

Locality development conforms most closely to the consensus model of society and is thus associated with traditional community development. It emphasizes self-help and concerted local action by the overall community. Implementation and change are seen as matters of communication among leaders and citizens (and planners) to gain an understanding of what needs to be done. Thus, the practitioner serves the **process** of facilitation of communications and interactions among all concerned. As stated by Rothman,

> The basic change strategy involves getting a broad cross section of people involved in studying and taking action on their problems. Consensus strategies are employed, involving small-group discussion and fostering communication among community subparts (class, ethnic,

Figure 8.3

Two Models of Community Organization and Implementation

PRACTICE VARIABLES	LOCALITY DEVELOPMENT	SOCIAL ACTION
Goal Categories of Community Action.	Developing community capacity and integration; self-help (process goals).	Change in power relationships and resource allocations; basic institutional change (task or process goals).
Assumptions Concerning Community Structure and Problem Conditions.	Lack of relationships and democratic problem-solving capacities; static community.	Disadvantaged populations, social injustice, inequity, unserved segments.
Basic Change Strategy	Involvement of citizens and leaders in identifying and solving their own problems.	Articulation and aggregation of issues, and organization of people to take action against power structure; demands on or take-over of larger system.
Characteristic Change Tactics and Techniques.	Consensus-building; communication among leaders and citizens; group processes.	Confrontation, direct action, advocacy; conflict or contest.
Salient Practitioner Roles.	Enabler-catalyst; coordinator; educator for problem-solving and democratic ethics.	Activist, advocate, agitator, broker, negotiator, partisan, politician.
Medium of Change	Manipulation of small, task-oriented groups; community meetings.	Manipulation of community groups, mass organizations and political processes.
Orientation Toward Power Structure.	Collaboration: leaders and citizens working in a common venture.	Confrontation: power structure as target of action, oppressors to be coerced or overturned.
Boundary of Constituency or Client System.	Total geographic community as beneficiary and participants.	Community segment as collaborators and participants.
Assumptions Regarding Interests of Community Sub-Parts.	Common interests or reconcilable differences; variable sum game.	Conflicting interests which are not easily reconcilable; zero sum game.

*Adapted from Rothman (1974), Figure 1.1. The Cox et al. reader (1974) is based on Rothman's categories and includes an extensive treatment of the models.

and so forth). The practitioner . . . is especially skilled in manipulating and guiding small-group interaction. (Rothman, 1974, p. 34.)

Locality development thus assumes that the community is comprised of people who share values and orientations, and who subscribe to democratic processes of decisionmaking and control. President Lyndon Johnson's favorite phrase, "Come let us reason together," typifies this model.

The contrasting approach, **social action**, also emphasizes grassroots strategies, but it views the community as a hierarchy of privilege and power. The task, therefore, is to confront the community with a show of force to convince the authorities that change is in order. Rothman puts it this way:

The basic change strategy involves crystallizing issues and organizing indigenous populations to take action on their own behalf against enemy targets. Change tactics often include conflict techniques, such as confrontation and direct action--rallies, marches, boycotts (as well as "hard-nosed" bargaining). The practitioner . . . is skilled in the manipulation of mass organizations and political processes. (Rothman, 1974, p. 35)

The fundamental difference between the two approaches is very clear: consensus vs. conflict. The overall goal of locality development is to enhance the relationship between the community power structure and its citizens. The means to this end is consensus-building through involvement of leaders and citizens in identifying and solving their problems. Consensus-building through small groups leads to increased well-being for the total community. This approach assumes that all parties have, or can come to have, common interests, and any differences are reconcilable through rational discussion and interaction.

The overall goal of social action, on the other hand, is to redress an imbalance of power between dominant and minority groups, and to gain allocations of resources for a segment or disadvantaged group. This model presumes that the power structure will not give up its benefits and privileges willingly. Thus, it is necessary to confront the power structure with a demonstration of popular power to convince it to change. As with advocacy planning, the social action model is appropriate where a community segment or disadvantaged group is involved. Locality development would be used where the entire community must, or could, be engaged to address a common need or problem. These two "faces" of grassroots action present most clearly the implications of the two models of society for community practice.

Two Models of Management

Management pervades systems and organizations. It provides the direction and control without which systems would fall apart. For our purposes, however, we will focus on those activities which are essential to ongoing operations. The term is derived from the French, **menage,** meaning "housekeeping." Thus, management is the organization and conduct of the affairs of a household, or an organization.

Frederick Winslow Taylor is credited with originating the modern practice of "scientific management" in 1895. Taylor recognized that, despite the authority and power of managers, workers really decided what got done. His approach was to create efficiencies and uniformity in the behavior of line-level workers, and thus to improve the efficiency of the organization. Recognition by more recent scholars of the "human" side of management led to behavioral and human relations approaches. Consider some definitions from the field:

> **Management is knowing exactly what you want men to do, and then seeing that they do it in the best and cheapest way.**
> **-Frederick W. Taylor.**

> The art of "getting things done" [and] . . . the manner in which the decisions and behavior of [production level] employees are influenced within and by the organization.
> -Herbert A. Simon

We allocate tasks, delegate authority, channel communication, and find some way of co-ordinating all that has been divided up and parceled out.
                                                                        —Philip Selznick

COORDINATING THE COLLECTIVE ACTIVITIES OF A GROUP OF INDIVIDUALS TOWARD A SET OF GOALS.
                                                                        —Rogers & McIntire

the problem solving or decision making segment of an organization.
                                                                        —Stanley Young

Managers are to an organization as the mind is to a person.
                                                                        —Franklin G. Moore

performance of the task of designing, predicting the results of, providing the resources for, and controlling an integrated human-group activity, the related physical facilities and the interrelationships between these two when the activity concerns the creation and distribution of goods or services to meet an external objective.
                                                                        —Marvin E. Mundel

While engineers are concerned with physical and chemical reactions, managers are concerned with the interactions of men.
                                                                        —Sir Geoffery Vickers

GETTING THINGS DONE THROUGH (OR BY) OTHERS.
                                                                        —Bertram M. Gross

Management thus involves the direction and control of how the units of a system are organized and how they interact. Management entails both the external and the internal relationships which are vital to the operation of a system.

Management is generally classified into three levels: top management, middle management, and lower management. **Top management** is concerned with the overall organization or system as a whole. Directors, secretaries, board chairmen, presidents and vice presidents, city managers and executive directors fall into this category. **Middle management** refers to several levels of managers that have responsibility for sections or functional areas. Bureau chiefs, office directors, budget and personnel managers, program heads and department managers of all kinds qualify. These are frequently the people for whom the phrase "bureaucrat" is most apt. **Lower management,** or first-level management, is made up of supervisors, unit directors, foremen, and other white-collar employees who are most directly in charge of day-to-day operations. These team leaders and supervisors have responsibility for assuring that production and delivery-level staff perform according to regulations and procedures.

At each level, managers are responsible for receiving messages and resources from upper levels, for communicating information and directions to lower levels, and for communicating information on performance and problems back up the chain of command. Top management, likewise, performs these roles with the external environment, seeking direction and resources for system survival and making policies and giving directions for subsystem operations.

We should also note that a distinction exists between **line** and **staff** personnel. "Line" workers are responsible most directly for the service or product of the organization. As such, the chain of authority extends directly from the top leadership directly to the delivery or production-level worker. "Staff" personnel are essential to the organization, and are indirectly related to the product. They provide the advisory, research, analysis and development roles which inform leadership of factors associated with past, present and future decisions. Staff personnel provide the policy research, planning, legal, implementation and training functions. Line personnel create the product and deliver the services of the organization. Thus, management is concerned with the direction and control of all units, in particular with the efficiency and effectiveness of line personnel; it also involves the activities used to promote efficient, effective, and accountable action by a system or organization.

Ideal Types: Bureaucratic Management and Management of Innovation

The management process originated by Frederick Winslow Taylor sounds highly rational and scientific. And most of the literature on modern management and public administration follows the rational-comprehensive model. Recent studies of both the management of community organizations and large corporations which experienced innovation and growth in a time of recession have led to examination of what successful managers actually do, compared to what the rationalist approach would say they ought to do. This emerging debate in the field provides an opportunity to develop ideal type models in this area to parallel the preceding sections.

One model will be called the **bureaucratic management,** or the institutional management approach--to reflect the consensus model of society; and the other will be labeled **management of innovation,** or the intuitive management approach--to reflect the conflict model of society.* Figure 8.4 identifies characteristics of the two approaches.

Bureaucratic management tends to occur in well-established organizations which are accepted in the community. Emphasis is on dealing with **routine operations and control of ongoing activities.** Thus, budgeting, personnel administration, supply logistics and supervision of line personnel predominate. Professionalism, efficiency and quantity are valued. Change is seen as being incremental; for example, five percent a year. Operations are based on written regulations and procedures. Administrative and management personnel have well-established roles, and the line-staff distinction is clear. Established relationships with environmental organizations make for comparatively "placid" interorganizational interactions.

Several labels are applied to the models due to the emerging nature of the approaches; no one label has "caught on" at this time. In fact, "intuitive management" is another term which is being applied to our second model.

273

Figure 8.4

Two Models of Management

PRACTICE VARIABLES	BUREAUCRATIC MANAGEMENT	MANAGEMENT OF INNOVATION
Goal Categories of Community Action.	Routine procedures and operations; status quo. Maintenance of existing organizational resources (task goals);	or, Adaptation to new environmental conditions (task and process goals.)
Assumptions Concerning Community Structure and Problem Conditions.	Organization well-established. Need to identify inefficient sub-units.	Organization is not well-established, or existence is threatened. need to gain support or acceptance in the community.
Basic Change Strategy	Change internal operations; systems improvement; rational-technical analysis.	Change the environment; systems design; interactive adjustment to environmental conditions, networking.
Characteristic Change Tactics and Techniques.	Authoritative direction; bureaucratic control.	Constituency-Building; campaign or contest.
Salient Practitioner Roles.	Budgeting, systems analysis, personnel management, information systems, accounting.	Negotiation (politician), grant and contract management, deemphasis on budgeting, etc. of routine and technical aspects of administration.
Medium of Change	Manipulation of formal organizations; rational systems analysis concerning sub-units.	manipulation of community processes and formal organizations; interactional processes concerning environmental actors.
Orientation Toward Power Structure.	Instrumental--a part of power structure. Power structure as employer.	Contention--power structure as target for acquisition of resources and power.
Boundary of Constituency or Client System.	Total community or community sub-system, or organization as subject.	New or threatened organization, sub-system or segment as constituency or collaborator.
Assumptions Regarding Interests of Community Sub-Parts.	Dominant interests are supportive. Consensus or competition perspective. Mnagement and/or application of authority is required.	Conflicting interests challenge the organization from without. Need to establish space in the interorganizational domain. Conflict perspctive--seeking authority, resources and power.

Management of innovation, or charismatic management, is most appropriate for new or changing organizations, and for situations where significant challenges from the environment occur. Emphasis is on goal-setting and the control and direction of program or system design. Tactics require acquisitive operations to obtain resources, to develop a constituency, and **to establish a place in the organizational domain.** Change of the organization and its place in the community is the immediate goal of this model. A more collegial, "flat" organizational structure is typical; and administrative, management and other roles are often blurred and/or staff is multifunctional. More interpersonal, interactive and face-to-face relationships exist. Emphasis is more on service to a target group, quality of the product, and perceived effectiveness. Establishment of relationships in the interorganizational domain and securing resources are major challenges.

Bureaucratic management conforms most closely to what van Gigch calls the "system improvement" approach; and management of innovation uses a "systems design" perspective. The former tends to be **introspective,** looking inward for problems in subunits or processes. The emphasis of bureaucratic management is thus on the status quo within the broader community system. Organizations characterized by this approach have difficulty in responding to change. The latter tends to be **extrospective,** concerned with the role of the organization in the broader community. As such, it is open to questioning its goals and to initiating conflict with community organizations. This approach is most appropriate for organizations which are faced with major challenges from the environment, and those that desire to create change.

Consequently, the orientation of the bureaucratic management model to the **power structure** is **instrumental.** This means that the organization is part of the existing power structure and/or is well established in the interorganizational network. While most likely the organization is in a competitive relationship with others, the total community status quo is supported and supportive. This consensus model situation contrasts sharply with that of management of innovation where a new or threatened organization is in **contention** with the status quo for **authority, resources and power.** In the former, we would expect dominant interests to be relatively supportive. Bureaucratic management can thus focus inward to

275

improve its efficiency in producing products or services. Hence, the relationship of this model to the consensus model of society. In the latter situation, attention must be given to survival and change, which requires a conflict model of action.

The two management models complete our repertoire of ideal type models of community engagement. The six models, or approaches to change, provide a basis for a conceptual understanding of the major aspects of policymaking and implementation. The development and selection of optional courses of action, strategies, provide a proactive basis on which to base present actions and to anticipate future decisions. Transformation of a plan from idea to action requires careful consideration of the methods of engagement of both citizens and leaders in a community. Finally, the management of the process requires skill and wisdom in getting things done by, or through, others. Each of the stages-- planning, implementation and management--is essential to the continued existence of specific programs and systems, and for the overall network of community systems and human services. We find it appropriate, therefore, to devote the last few sections of the book to a discussion of the interrelation of the models in the real world.

Situational Relativity: Mixing Strategies in the Real World

Strategies are not executed in isolation, and only rarely is the pure form appropriate in real-world situations. Rather, strategies should be "mixed and phased" as appropriate for specific scenarios. Figure 8.5 presents a refinement of Stockdale's framework for the analysis of change strategies at the community level. (Stockdale, 1976) Interrelationships among strategies can be made on both horizontal (left-right) and vertical (up-down) dimensions. This chart allows us to compare similarities and differences among the strategies on the several practice variables.

On the **horizontal** dimension, the more rational-technical and task-oriented strategies appear on the left. Institutional (bureaucratic) management and the two planning strategies tend to be technological and office-bound, relying more on analyses, reports, and the like, than the other approaches. Locality development, social

Figure 8.5

Strategies of Change

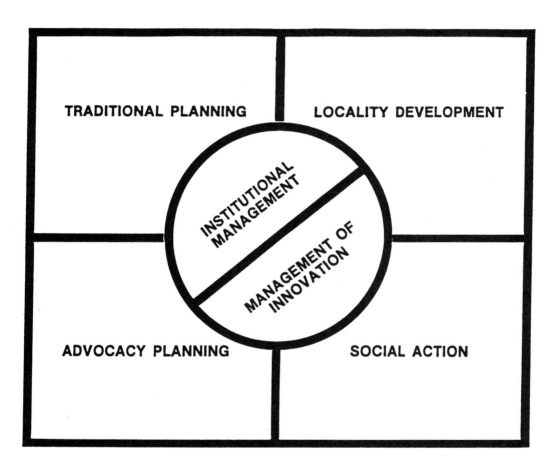

action and management of innovation place more emphasis on community processes and interactions--they can be said to be more interpersonal and community-bound.

On the **vertical** dimension, the strategies depicted at the top of the chart tend to have a consensus-based approach to change and the strategies on the bottom are oriented to the conflict model. Thus, social action, advocacy planning and management of innovation generally address a community segment or subpopulation, and are most likely to use conflict and contest strategies. Locality development, traditional planning and bureaucratic management tend to view the overall community as their constituency and, in turn, to rely on collaborative strategies.

Now, consider the strategies in relation to our model of the policymaking process--the political system. The strategies on the **top** of the chart tend to be most appropriate for use by those in power--the authorities--and those who collaborate with the power structure. The strategies on the **bottom** are more appropriate for those not in power but who are seeking change by the authorities, and those who are seeking a role in the power structure. The goal of these latter strategies is to make **effective demands** on the authorities. For example, a city planner may devise a nutrition program for the city health department. He/she works for and presents the plan to the city authorities. A neighborhood planner, however, in working for a specific subarea may prepare a nutrition plan which is directed to convincing the city authorities to alter their plan to provide more or different services to the the neighborhood. The former involves a process **within** the power structure to decide what actions to take in the overall community. The latter involves a process **external to** the power structure directed to creating an **input** to the deliberations of the city authorities.

The example above illustrates the differences in focus of the two models, and it raises the issue of boundaries and system levels. Note that if the city planner is preparing a plan to be presented to higher authority--state or federal levels, for example--there is a completely different role: the perspective changes. (**"Where you stand depends upon where you sit."**) Likewise, a neighborhood planner working with his/her own local funds on a neighborhood plan is in a service allocation, not a resource acquisition, role. Focus thus shifts to relationships with the immediate community, rather than convincing an external power structure to support the plan.

278

The chart also enables us to consider compatibilities between strategies and the possibility of shifting from one to another. **Adjacent strategies,** those that share a common boundary on the chart, can be seen as a continuum of possible actions. In action situations, shifting from one strategy to another may be appropriate. (Stockdale, 1976) An advocacy planner, for example, if successful in convincing the authorities that a plan (for a segment) is good for the entire community, may find the plan transformed into a community-wide "traditional planning" document. Similarly, if a group using locality development as a strategy encounters resistance from the authorities, it may find itself in a social action situation. Understanding these interactions is important for the community practitioner for it establishes a broad range of strategies in his/her repertoire (instead of just six). Most importantly, this discussion emphasizes the interactive nature of community action and change. If strategies are not modified to reflect changing community and environmental conditions, they will rapidly become obsolete and fail.

Note, too, that the two management strategies are placed on a diagonal to the other four. This arrangement recognizes the fact that bureaucratic, or institutional, management is most generally associated with the more technical and/or total community strategies: locality development, traditional planning and advocacy planning. Recall also that management of innovation is appropriate both for new organizations, for those dealing with a segment, and for existing organizations which are facing an external challenge. Thus, a new organization using a locality development strategy would be likely to choose management of innovation; and we would expect a shift toward bureaucratic management as the organization becomes established in the community. Similarly, a traditional planning organization using bureaucratic management, when faced with funding cuts from external authorities, could be expected to shift to an advocacy planning mode and to utilize management of innovation strategies. Note, too, that social action does not share a boundary with institutional management and traditional planning; and traditional planning does not share a boundary with mangement of innovation and social action. These pairings tend to be unlikely as explained below.

Another principle which is illustrated on Figure 8.5 is that **nonadjacent strategies,** those on a diagonal across from each other, tend to be **incompatible.** The most conflict-oriented strategy, social action, would tend to be incompatible with the most consensus-oriented strategies of traditional planning and bureaucratic management. While variations across all dimensions of the six models should be available as options for every action situation, it should be recognized that successful mixing and phasing of the nonadjacent approaches are less likely. Likewise, locality development, which uses group, consensus-oriented approaches to the overall community, and advocacy planning, which emphasizes rational-technical conflict approaches for a community segment would tend to be incompatible. If environmental conditions or organizational goals change, however, and an organization using a locality development approach should find itself in a social action relationship with the authorities, then advocacy planning enters as a more likely complementary strategy. Understanding these interrelationships is important to the community professional, for aspects of planning, organizing-implementation and management exist in every organization, and they occur on a broader community basis as well. A particular unit or program may adopt one model as the dominant, overall strategy; the other models then become available as possible tactics and/or ways of addressing the various aspects of guiding and operating the ongoing program or system. Aspects of these latter relationships are examined in the next section.

A Hierarchical View of the Six Strategies

The six models have been presented as ideal types in order to categorize, analyze and explain their characteristics. In practice, community organizations and programs use approximations or mixtures of the pure types. Furthermore, any one organization or program has a need to address all aspects of the programming model explicated in the previous chapter. Figure 8.6 depicts the strategies in a manner which facilitates exploration of additional dimensions of selection and employment.

The chart is arranged in a pyramid which is suggestive of the levels of the policymaking system: community, regime and

Figure 8.6

Strategies and Levels of Change

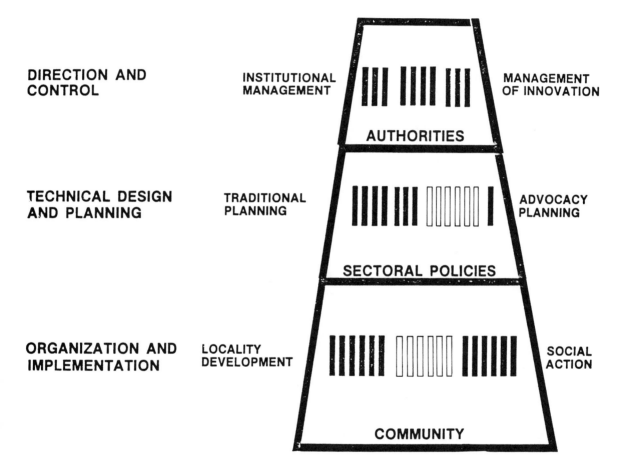

**DIRECTION AND
CONTROL**

INSTITUTIONAL
MANAGEMENT

MANAGEMENT
OF INNOVATION

AUTHORITIES

**TECHNICAL DESIGN
AND PLANNING**

TRADITIONAL
PLANNING

ADVOCACY
PLANNING

SECTORAL POLICIES

**ORGANIZATION AND
IMPLEMENTATION**

LOCALITY
DEVELOPMENT

SOCIAL
ACTION

COMMUNITY

authorities. **Community** is where needs and problems occur and where the outputs and impacts of policies and programs are felt. Interests are articulated and aggregated at this level; and this is where programs must be implemented. Thus, as indicated in the chart, the organizing and implementation strategies would be most dominant here. At the intermediate level, where the staff planning and administrative roles tend to occur, we find the planning strategies. The development of data to support decisons and options for dealing with problems and needs, for evaluating impact, and for designing new approaches tend to occur at this level. Finally, the authorities are responsible for the overall direction and control of the organization, program or system.

Consider these levels in light of the "system within system" principle. The pyramid can be seen to apply at all levels of a community system: within a specific program, the relationship of a program to the environment, and in the overall community. A neighborhood mental health clinic, for example, might well have grassroots strategies involving consultation and education for local self-help. It would, nevertheless, need to have planning and management functions performed in the organization. Direct line staff at the street-level would tend to be organizationally at a lower level than staff planners and program managers. The entire organization, however, would be at a "lower" level in the vertical hierarchy of the overall community than a city-level mental health planning agency. The latter, in turn, would be subordinate to the city manager and council. Constant attention to the boundaries of inquiry and the focal system is necessary to avoid misdirection and misunderstanding. A principle of "situational relativity" could be said to apply to this phenomenon: the type of strategy which is most important changes with the situation in the community-organizational hierarchy.

Note, too, that the strategies are arranged to suggest a continuum at each level. Grassroots **organizing and implementation** strategies range from locality development to pure social action. **Planning** strategies vary from idealized traditional planning to advocacy planning. **Management** strategies span a continuum from an ideal-type bureaucratic management to management of innovation.

Any organization has a full range of strategies on which to draw to pursue its goals and to respond to changing environmental conditions. Consider the situation of a neighborhood group which has the support of some, but not all, of the authorities for a community-wide transportation program for the aged. The group could be considered to be in a situation calling for a locality development strategy based on the community-wide character of the issue. On the other hand, there are two segmental characteristics to the constituency (neighborhood and an elderly quasi-group) which would suggest a social action approach. The organization would be wise to use different tactics in working with neighborhood citizens and proponents of the aged throughout the community than with the opposing authorities and their supporters.

A comparable "mixed strategy" situation would exist in a scenario in which traditional planners in a justice agency find opposition in management circles or among community residents. It would be appropriate to consider some advocacy planning practices to work with community groups and to convince the authorities of the validity of the plans. At the highest level, an established organization using a bureaucratic management model might be confronted with opposition in the community or budget cuts from external funding sources; the need to revise its strategy to use some management of innovation, and perhaps a bit of advocacy planning, is apparent.

Finally, note that the two sides of the pyramid conform generally to the primary models of society. The strategies on the left side tend to be consonant with the **consensus model** and the strategies on the right side conform to the principles of the **conflict model**. This brings us full circle. We have explored approaches which allow the interrelation of the general model of the policymaking process, fundamental paradigms of Western philosophy and social thought, the overall programming model for community and human services, and models of action strategies. These concepts, processes and models occur in community systems; they are essential to the formulation and implementation of policies to establish, direct and regulate community systems and human services.

Some Concluding Thoughts:
The Unit and the Unity

Reality is a complex web of interactions--of system within system within system. Simultaneous and parallel processes occur throughout human systems, creating conflict and stress at every point; and at every point we find cohesion--whether from shared values or from constraint. The written word, however, requires a linear process to present ideas in a rational train of thought. Constant reiteration of the relationships among ideas and concepts presented herein and attention to their application in communities have been directed to promoting an understanding of both the pieces and the overall picture.

We have offered a foundation for developing knowledge about the **units** of community systems, and for analysis of their role in **systems** and subsystems. A basis has been suggested for understanding the **unity** of units and subsystems as parts of larger wholes. Our knowledge currently is partial and highly disciplne-bound. As we gain more knowledge of the parts and their interactions, we can look forward to developing a fuller understanding of communities and change. We have emphasized the counterposition of values and actions, of ideas and reality, and of consensus and conflict. It is our hope that, as you develop an analytical understanding of the many facets of community and human development, you will also seek their synthesis into a more complete, useful understanding of the future we all are creating.

Drew Hyman
Joe A. Miller

University Park, Pa.
A.D. 1985

Chapter VIII

REFERENCES

Alinsky, Saul D. "Of Means and Ends." **Rules for Radicals.** N. Y.: Random House, Inc., 1971.

Altshuler, Alan. "The Goals of Comprehensive Planning." in Faludi, op. cit., 1973, pp. 193-210.

Banfield, Edward C. "Politics, Planning and the Public Interest," in Fred M. Cox et al., **Strategies of Community Organization.** Itasca, Ill.: F. E. Peacock Publishers, Inc., 2nd Ed., 1974, pp. 307-320.

Caiden, Gerald E. "Implementation--The Achilles Heel of Administrative Reform." in Arne F. Leemans, **The Management of Change in Government.** The Netherlands: The Hague, 1976.

Cox, Fred M., John L. Erlich, Jack Rothman and John E. Tropman, eds. **Strategies of Community Organization.** Itasca, Ill.: F. E. Peacock Publishers, Inc., 1974.

Dahl, Robert A. "The Politics of Planning." **International Social Science Journal.** 11:3, 1959.

Dror, Yehezkel. "The Planning Process." in Faludi, op. cit., 1973, pp. 329-336. Faludi, Andreas. **A Reader in Planning Theory.** N. Y.: Pergamon Press, 1973.

Glass, Ruth. "The Evaluation of Planning." in Andreas Faludi, **A Reader in Planning Theory.** N. Y.: Pergamon Press, 1973, pp. 45-68.

Gross, Bertram M. **Organizations and Their Managing.** N. Y.: The Free Press, 1964.

Hunter, Floyd, Ruth Connor Schaffer, and Cecil G. Sheps. **Community Power Structure.** Chapel Hill: University of North Carolina Press, 1956, p. 241.

Lindeman, Eduard C. **The Community.** N. Y.: The Association Press, 1921, p. 139.

McDonald, John. **Strategy in Poker, Business & War.** N. Y.: W. W. Norton & Co., Inc., 1950.

Moore, Franklin G. **The Management of Organizations.** N. Y.: John Wiley & Sons, 1982, p. 6.

Mundel, Marvin E. **A Conceptual Framework for the Management Sciences.** N. Y.: McGraw-hill Book Co., 1967, p. 4.

Newman, William H. **Administrative Action.** N. Y.: Pitman Publishing Co., 1958.

Rogers, Rolf E., and Robert H. Mcintire. **Organization and Management Theory.** N. Y.: John Wiley & Sons, 1983.

Ross, Murray G. **Community Organization Thory and Practice.** N. Y.: Harper and Row, 1955, p. 61.

Rothman, Jack. "Three Models of Community Organization Practice." in Cox et al., **op. cit.,** p. 20-36.

Selznick, Philip. "Leadership in Administration," in Robert T. Golembiewski, Frank Gibson and Geoffrey Y. Cornog, **Public Administration.** Chicago, Ill.: Rand-McNally, 1966, p. 412-419.

Simon, Herbert A. **Administrative Behavior.** N. Y.: The MacMillan Co., 1948.

Steiner, Jesse F. **Community Organization.** rev. ed. N. Y.: The Century Co., 1930.

Stockdale, Jerry D. "Community Organization Practice: An Elaboration of Rothman's Typology." **Sociology and Social Welfare,** 3, May 1976, 541-551.

Taylor, Frederick W. **Shop Management.** N. Y.: Harper & Bros, 1911, p. 21.

United Nations. **Special Study on Social Conditions in Non-Self-Governing Territories.** N. Y.: The United Nations, 1956.

Vickers, Geoffrey. **Towards a Sociology of Management.** N. Y.: Basic Books, 1967, p. 9.

Williams, Walter. **The Implementation Perspective.** Los Angeles: The University of California Press, 1980.

Young, Stanley. **Management: A Systems Analysis.** Glenview, Ill.: Scott, Foresman and Co., 1966.

Zastrow, Charles. **The Practice of Social Work.** Homewood, Ill.: Dorsey Press, 1981.

INDEX